LANGLEY ADAMS LIBRARY

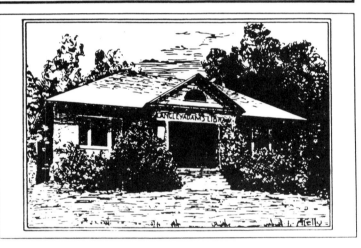

November 2002

A PARENT'S GUIDE TO ASPERGER SYNDROME AND HIGH-FUNCTIONING AUTISM

A Parent's Guide
to Asperger Syndrome
and High-Functioning Autism

*How to Meet the Challenges
and Help Your Child Thrive*

618.92

SALLY OZONOFF
GERALDINE DAWSON
JAMES McPARTLAND

The Guilford Press
New York   London

35.00

11-02

© 2002 The Guilford Press
A Division of Guilford Publications, Inc.
72 Spring Street, New York, NY 10012
www.guilford.com

Printed in the United States of America

This book is printed on acid-free paper.

Last digit is print number: 9   8   7   6   5   4   3   2   1

Library of Congress Cataloging-in-Publication Data

Ozonoff, Sally.
      A parent's guide to Asperger syndrome and high-functioning autism
    : how to meet the challenges and help your child thrive / Sally Ozonoff,
Geraldine Dawson, James McPartland.
          p. ; cm.
      Includes bibliographical references and index.
      ISBN 1-57230-531-2 (pbk. : alk. paper) — ISBN 1-57230-767-6
(hardcover : alk. paper)
      1. Asperger's syndrome—Popular works.   2. Autism—Popular
works.   [DNLM: 1. Asperger Syndrome.   2. Autistic Disorder.
3. Parenting.   WM 203.5 O99p 2002]   I. Dawson, Geraldine.
II. McPartland, James.   III. Title.
RJ506.A9 O98 2002
618.92′8982—dc21
                                                                2002005507

To my husband, Tom, who shares my passion
for autism, and my girls, Grace and Claire,
who tolerated the writing of this book when they
wanted to play

—S.O.

To my husband, Joseph, and daughter, Margaret
—G.D.

To my parents and greatest mentors, Rosemary
and Jim McPartland

—J.M.

CONTENTS

Contents

ACKNOWLEDGMENTS

The writing of this book would not have been possible without the parents and children who shared their stories, pain, hopes, and triumphs with me. I have learned far more from them than I have been able to give back. Thank you for letting me be a part of your lives at your bleakest moments and at your times of joy. I have learned so much from my mentors, Bruce Pennington, who taught me the science of autism; Sally Rogers, who taught me the art of autism; and Gary Mesibov, who immersed me in the culture of autism. I've never wanted to do anything else since these three introduced me to autism. Kitty Moore and Christine Benton of The Guilford Press helped greatly in the writing of this book and often knew what I wanted to say better than I did. I also thank my father, who instilled a love of words and taught me to write; my mother, who cooked many delicious meals so that I could write; my husband, who calmed me down; and my sweet girls, Grace and Claire, who danced, sang, played dress-up, and colored while I wrote.

—S.O.

I wish to gratefully acknowledge all I have learned from the children and parents with whom I have worked. Their experiences, feedback, and creative ideas have greatly influenced my thinking and practice over the years, and their perseverance, passion, and resilience are a constant source of inspiration for me. My colleagues and students at the University of Washington Autism Center have also been instrumental in the writing of this book, especially Felice Orlich, Kimberly Ryan, and Cathy Brock. I have very much enjoyed working with the staff at The Guilford Press, especially Seymour Weingarten, Kitty Moore, and Christine Benton; this book has very much benefited from their guidance and expertise. Finally, I wish to express heartfelt appreciation for the unwavering love and support I receive from my husband, Joseph, and my children, Christopher and Margaret. Without their support, my work would not be possible.

—G.D.

I feel fortunate to have interacted with so many devoted parents and wonderful children within the autism community. My contributions to this text represent the synthesis of the lessons I have learned from you, and I thank you for working with me. It has been enjoyable and educational to collaborate with my coauthors on this project, as well as the staff at The Guilford Press. I am also grateful to those who have taught me about autism, most notably, Geraldine Dawson, Felice Orlich, and Julie Osterling. I am most thankful for the support of my fiancée, Tara, and her tolerance for the sound of typing in the middle of the night.

—J.M.

PART I

Understanding Asperger Syndrome and High-Functioning Autism

CHAPTER 1

....

*What Are Asperger Syndrome
and High-Functioning Autism?*

Joseph had always seemed like a brilliant child. He began talking before his first birthday, much earlier than his older sister and brother. He expressed himself in an adult way and was always very polite. When his mother offered to buy him a treat at the movies, for example, Joseph said, "No, thank you, M&M's are not my preferred mode of snacking." He showed a very early interest in letters and by 18 months could recite the whole alphabet. He taught himself to read before his third birthday. Joseph wasn't much interested in typical toys, like balls and bicycles, preferring instead what his proud parents considered "grown-up" pursuits, like geography and science. Starting at age 2, he spent many hours lying on the living-room floor, looking at maps in the family's world atlas. By age 5, he could name anywhere in the world from a description of its geographical location ("What is the northern-most coastal city in Brazil?"). Just as his parents suspected, Joseph *is* brilliant. He also has Asperger syndrome.

Nine-year-old Seth was playing video games in the family room while his mother bustled about the house cleaning up for the guests who would soon arrive. As she climbed a stepladder in the living room to change a lightbulb, she lost her balance and fell backward. While she lay on the floor gasping for breath, Seth walked by on his way to the

3

kitchen for a snack, stepped over her, and said "Hi, Mom." Seth has high-functioning autism.

Clint turns 30 soon. He graduated from college with a degree in engineering, lives in an apartment in a nice section of town, recently bought a used car, and enjoys going to the movies. He is troubled, however, by his difficulty finding and keeping a job. Time and again, supervisors get frustrated by his slow work pace and difficulty getting along with coworkers. Clint gets stuck on details and finds it hard to set goals that eventually lead to completion of projects. After finishing a seasonal job cleaning hotel rooms at a ski resort, he tells prospective employers that he was "let go" without realizing that this term means "fired" to most people. Unable to find work for months, he visits a vocational counselor, who suggests a psychological evaluation. Testing reveals that Clint has high-functioning autism, which was never diagnosed.

Lauren is a teenager with the looks of a model. Despite this, she has no friends, nor does she seem particularly interested in having any. She still loves Barbie dolls at age 17 and collects every new model and outfit that comes on the market. At school, Lauren often appears to be daydreaming; when directions are given to the class, she does not respond as she sits smiling and occasionally talking softly to herself. Despite this, she is a straight-A student who excels in mathematics and physics. When other kids greet her in the hallways, she sometimes does not notice and other times looks away while mumbling a quick "Hi." Now the school psychologist has mentioned to Lauren's parents that she may have high-functioning autism or Asperger syndrome. How could their beautiful, perfect daughter have something like *autism*? her distraught parents wonder. And what on earth is Asperger syndrome?

Joseph, Seth, Clint, and Lauren all have what doctors now call *high-functioning autism spectrum disorders*. If your child resembles them in any way, you may have heard the names of the conditions falling under the autism spectrum umbrella: high-functioning autism and Asperger syndrome. And you probably have a million questions about them, just as Lauren's parents did: What are these conditions? What is the difference between them? What causes them? How could my unique and interesting child, who has so many strengths, also have such difficulties? What will the future bring for him or her, and us? This book will answer these questions and many more. In this chapter we define some important terms to help you decide if this book is relevant for you and whether it may help the person in your life who has similar strengths and similar challenges. We'll also tell you what we know about who has these disorders and what the future may bring to these children and their families.

The word *autism* was coined from the Greek word *autos,* meaning self. The term was first used to describe behavior in 1943 by Leo Kanner, a child psychiatrist at Johns Hopkins University in Baltimore. In his landmark paper, Dr. Kanner described 11 children who showed little interest in other people, insisted on routines, and displayed unusual body movements, like flapping their hands. Many of the children could talk: some could name things in their environment, others could count or say the alphabet, still others could recite whole books, word for word, from memory. However, they rarely used their speech to communicate with others. The children had a variety of learning problems in addition to their unusual behaviors.

For many years after Dr. Kanner's initial description, only those children whose behaviors were very similar in type and severity to those of the original cases were diagnosed with autism. Slowly, however, we began to recognize that autism has a wide variety of faces and can be found in children with good communication skills, who are of normal intelligence, who have few learning problems, and who show milder versions of the behaviors Dr. Kanner described. These are the so-called *high-functioning* individuals; this term has been defined in different ways but generally means having normal intelligence and a fairly good command of language. We now know that autism is not a narrowly defined condition, but rather a spectrum that varies in severity from the classic picture described by Leo Kanner to milder variants associated with good language and cognitive (thinking) skills. For this reason, we now use the term *autism spectrum disorders.* The subject of this book is high-functioning autism spectrum disorders.

Good language and cognitive skills mean that many children with these disorders, like Joseph and Lauren, do just fine in school and often get along well with adults. But in other ways, Joseph's unusual behaviors make life challenging. Joseph's intense interests often disrupt family activities; his parents are often not able to persuade him to leave his science projects to use the bathroom or come to the dinner table. On a recent trip to Disneyland, he insisted on bringing his globe, which had to be transported in a baby stroller throughout the park. Joseph's professor-like speech makes him stand out among his peers, who delight in teasing him and never accept his invitations to come over and play. Joseph has begun to make negative comments about himself ("I'm a geek"), and his parents worry about depression. Lauren, on the other hand, doesn't seem to mind being virtually friendless, but her parents are deeply saddened by her social isolation and the life that she is missing out on. Her mother bought her a dress for the junior prom, but Lauren refused to go; her mother spent the evening crying. Clint certainly has the intelligence to be successful, but his social awkwardness and blunt comments to coworkers ("Just get off your behind and do it") mean that he has never kept a job for longer than a few weeks. He is also underemployed: despite a degree in engineering, Clint has held a variety of manual labor and store clerk positions. And Seth illustrates one of the most far-reaching problems that people with high-functioning autism spectrum disorders have: difficulty with the kind of close, empathic relationships that are, in some ways, the essence of our humanity. Until her son was diagnosed with high-functioning autism, Seth's mother was convinced that she had in some way deeply damaged her son to cause such lack of regard for others and their feelings. When he was young, Seth would talk so loudly and behave so inappropriately in restaurants (for example, by taking food that appealed to him off other diners' plates) that the family was often asked to leave. Seth's mother remembered sympathizing with a neighbor whose daughter was in a wheelchair about the restrictions their children placed on their families. The neighbor listed several things her family couldn't do, such as go hiking together, and then asked in astonishment, "What can't *you* do?" And Seth's mother, taken aback, said, "Why, we can't do anything! Seth's behavior is so active and inappropriate in public, but he seems so normal, that everyone gives us terrible looks. It's just too hard on us, especially Seth's siblings." These conditions take a toll not only on the individuals who have them, but also on their families.

At about the same time that scientists began to realize that there was such a thing as high-functioning autism, Dr. Lorna Wing, an eminent British researcher at the Institute of Psychiatry in London, brought something called Asperger syndrome to the attention of the English-speaking world. Dr. Hans Asperger, an Austrian pediatrician, had first described Asperger syndrome in 1944, apparently without any knowledge of Leo Kanner's work. Because Asperger's paper was written in German and published during World War II, it was not widely read. Until Dr. Wing's paper was published in 1981, the condition remained virtually unknown in the United States and other non-German-speaking countries. In her paper, Dr. Wing summarized Asperger's original publication, but she also noted the similarities between Asperger syndrome and autism, raising for the first time a question that is still with us today: Are Asperger syndrome and autism the same disorder or two separate ones?

Because Asperger syndrome is in a sense only 20 years old, a relatively small amount of reliable scientific data has been collected on it. To date the research has found few differences between Asperger syndrome and high-functioning autism. This is not to suggest that there are no differences between the two disorders—though that is a matter of ongoing debate. There is, for example, a learning profile sometimes associated with Asperger syndrome that may occur less often in high-functioning autism. Chapter 2 goes into more detail on the distinctions between the two diagnoses. What is important to parents of children who may have one of these problems is that the two conditions present many of the same challenges and that similar treatments seem to help both disorders. Research suggests that what has been written about high-functioning autism (HFA) is relevant and applicable to Asperger syndrome (AS), so the practical guidance in this book will help those with either condition. In fact, we will use the term *AS-HFA* throughout this book to include *both* conditions, but will make it clear when any information is specifically relevant to only one diagnosis or the other.

Unfortunately, this does not mean that your child's doctor will use the same term that we use. Because there is still much professional disagreement about how autism, high-functioning autism, Asperger syndrome, and autism spectrum disorders fit together, a doctor who evaluates your child may use several terms. Complicating matters, some doctors will disagree with our view that high-functioning autism and Asperger syndrome are similar (more on this in Chapter 2). To make things even more confusing, there is also a condition called pervasive developmental disorder not otherwise specified (or PDDNOS for short)—something of a catchall label for children who show some of the characteristics of autism or Asperger syndrome, but cannot be fit neatly into either slot. As a parent, you will want to make sure that your child receives the most accurate diagnosis possible, but, in the case of these disorders, you need to be aware that precision may elude us for some time to come. What's important is that you feel confident that the picture you have of your child coincides with the picture your child's doctor offers and, regardless of the label, that the treatments suggested fit with your child's weaknesses and strengths.

If you are living with someone with Asperger syndrome or high-functioning autism, you probably wouldn't notice many differences between the conditions from day to day or from moment to moment. In fact, as you'll read in Chapter 2, the primary difference between the two conditions lies in children's behavior before they turn 3 years old. That difference can be discovered by a doctor who takes a careful history of your child's early development, but a doctor who observes your child for only a while, especially if he or she is of school age or older, would be hard-pressed to tell Asperger syndrome from high-functioning autism any more than a layperson could.

What High-Functioning Autism Spectrum Disorders Look Like

No one will display all the features that characterize these disorders; some individuals may exhibit only a few. Just as no two nonautistic people, even identical twins, are absolutely alike, no two individuals with Asperger syndrome or high-functioning autism behave in exactly the same way. All, however, have some difficulties interacting with other people and some odd or repetitive behaviors.

Problems with Social Interaction: Active but Odd

The essence of AS-HFA is difficulty with social interactions, although the striking social impairments of more classic autism, such as extreme remoteness and persistent avoidance of others, rarely appear. Some children, like Lauren, don't go out of their way to start conversations or interact with others but do respond if other people approach them. Other individuals show interest in people and enjoy their company; they may even want to join groups and make friends. However, their ability to do so successfully is limited by their difficulty knowing what to do or say in social situations. They may be awkward and unsure during interactions. They may give the impression that they are not interested in the person they are talking to because they don't follow the

A Few Key Terms—and What They Mean

pervasive developmental disorders (PDDs): a group of disorders characterized by delayed or abnormal development in many ("pervasive") aspects of development: social, communication, behavior, cognition, sometimes even motor skills. This term is synonymous with *autism spectrum disorders.*

pervasive developmental disorder not otherwise specified (PDDNOS): The child has some autistic-like behaviors, but does not meet the definition of either high-functioning autism or Asperger syndrome.

autism: the most common and typical of the PDDs, ranging in severity from those who are very handicapped (nonverbal, totally aloof, and highly repetitive) to those who are only mildly socially awkward, are slightly unusual in their conversational style, and have special interests.

high-functioning: having normal intelligence and a fairly good command of language.

The high-functioning autism spectrum disorders include:

high-functioning autism: The child fits the definition of autism but has normal cognitive and learning abilities. The child may initially have had difficulty acquiring language, but eventually was able to speak at a level close to what is expected for his or her age.

Asperger syndrome: The child is similar to those with high-functioning autism, but has fewer symptoms and had little or no difficulty developing language at the normal age.

Autism spectrum disorders affect up to 0.6% of the population, and two-thirds to three-quarters of those children appear to be high-functioning.

"rules" of social interaction. Most of us naturally know that we should look at the person we're talking to, smile, and nod occasionally to signify that we are paying attention. People with AS-HFA, however, don't seem to appreciate these unwritten rules of social engagement. Their behavior while out in public may sometimes be inappropriate or embarrassing when, in addition to failing to use these social niceties, they violate clear social conventions, such as keeping certain opinions to themselves or refraining from asking overly personal questions. It may indeed be true that your neighbor's upper arms look like "fat sausages," but this is information best kept to yourself.

People with high-functioning autism or Asperger syndrome often appear not to understand other people's feelings or points of view, which makes their social interactions even more difficult. Often these abilities, natural to the rest of us, are delayed or do not develop at all. Empathy usually begins emerging in infancy, when young children start to show an interest in and a concern about the feelings of others. It's not uncommon in daycare centers to see babies break into sympathetic wails when another infant cries or to see toddlers bring a toy or an adult to a crying child in an attempt to comfort their peer. Preschoolers are fascinated by the moods of others and often talk about friends being angry or sad. In their pretend play, young children enact scenes in which characters are sick or upset, grappling with understanding such states and how to respond to them.

In contrast, most children with AS-HFA have basic difficulty appreciating the emotions of others (and perhaps their own as well). As Seth's mother could attest, many children don't even notice when parents, siblings, or other children are hurt, sick, or sad, and even if they do they rarely offer comfort. Or they may horribly misunderstand others' feelings. One boy burst into laughter after his father fell down the stairs, tearing ligaments in his ankle. When his horrified mother asked why he was laughing, he explained, "Dad is jumping around and making funny faces like a clown." Clint described an interaction with a coworker who made "a strange face" after he told a joke. He didn't think much about it until later, when he saw a painting of a woman bearing the exact same facial expression. He showed the painting to his mother and asked how the woman felt. She said, "Offended, I think." Clint has felt bad about insulting his coworker ever since, but says, "If someone is insinuating something through their face or body, without being direct, I just can't grasp it." He has taken to studying art in the hopes that it will help him better understand people.

While they often establish warm, loving relationships and secure bonds with parents, siblings, and understanding adults, most, if not all, individuals with AS-HFA experience difficulty relating to peers of approximately the same age. Some children are teased or bullied, others are ignored by kids, and still others, like Lauren, seem perfectly content with no friends. A few children develop friendships that revolve around shared interests (such as video games), but rarely play anything else together, and the interaction stops when the activity ends. There is usually little of the sharing of secrets and reliance on each other for support that typically develop between friends during the middle childhood years. Many children with autism spectrum disorders report feeling lonely and socially isolated because of such peer difficulties. They are hurt by teasing and often unaware of their unusual behavior or social response that may contribute to the situation. In later childhood or adolescence, they often become painfully aware of their differences from others and their inability to understand the fundamentals of interaction that others accomplish naturally. One teen stated, "I know I'm supposed to look people in the eye—my parents are constantly reminding me—but it doesn't help me understand what they think or feel, so I just don't do it." This can lead to low self-esteem and low self-confidence that, in a vicious cycle, perpetuate the problems. As the child loses hope of social success, he or she gives up trying to interact with others. This only increases social isolation, which may further compound the awkwardness or outright oddity of the child's social behavior. In the most extreme cases, the cycle may lead to serious bouts of depression that require treatment.

Communication: Eloquent but Inarticulate

In addition to social difficulties, autism spectrum disorders usually involve communication problems. In fact, the most prominent feature of classic autism, at least in the minds of most people, is the inability to speak. What is less well understood is that even those with Asperger syndrome and high-functioning autism experience some difficulties with communication. This, it turns out, is one of the most confusing parts of the diagnostic puzzle and often leads to misdiagnoses when the child is young. You may have had autism raised as a possibility at some point in your child's life, only to have it "ruled out" or be told later that he or she couldn't possibly be autistic because the child speaks so well. Indeed, it is part of the definition of Asperger syndrome that language be fluent, not only at the age the child is seen for evaluation, but even at ages 2 and 3. A smaller, but not insignificant, number of children with high-functioning autism begin talking early and soon speak articulately in a manner that seems advanced. Parents may first believe their child is gifted based on his or her precocious language skills. Yet there are virtually always differences in the *way* language is used, particularly in social contexts, that can cause problems. The child, adolescent, or adult with AS-HFA may dominate conversations, talking on and on without giving others the chance to say anything. The pedantic or overly formal manner of speaking that Joseph uses is common in both Asperger syndrome and high-functioning autism. At age 7, Joseph begins many statements the way a professor might, saying, "Actually . . . " or "I do believe. . . . " He has a vast vocabulary and loves to use unusual words—the bigger the better. When asked his favorite color, he pointed to a yellow balloon and said with a smile "chartreuse." Clint defines terms that don't need defining. He readily tells people that he is autistic, hastening to add, "Autistic is the adjective for the noun autism" as if we would not know what the word meant without this explanation. While there is nothing technically wrong with phrasing things so formally, it certainly makes Clint and Joseph stand out from their peers and often makes them the target of teasing. Joseph's mother likens his speech patterns to someone who speaks English as a second language: other people can figure out what he is trying to say, but the way he phrases even simple statements makes it seem as if English is not his native tongue.

Some children with AS-HFA memorize things that other people say (or phrases or dialogue from videos and books) and then incorporate them into their own speech. This memorized speech is called *delayed echolalia* and, while idiosyncratic, does indicate that the child has a well-developed verbal memory. Sometimes the echoed phrases are used in context and make sense, as when Joseph exclaimed, "Oh no, it's my worst nightmare!" (dialogue from a Disney movie) after spilling milk on one of his maps. Other times, the link between the phrase and the context is less clear. Seth's mother reported that as a small child he would say "He's a happy man right there" whenever he put on or took off a hat. For years, she and Seth's dad had no idea where this comment came from or what it meant. Then one day they happened to be watching an old golf video they had taped several years earlier. They were astounded to see one of the golfers make a hole-in-one and then tip his cap to the audience as the announcer said, "He's a happy man right there." Seth had associated this phrase with hats, and the two remained linked in his mind, although the phrase made little sense to others and didn't help him communicate his wants or needs.

Another communication problem for children with AS-HFA is their *literal interpretation* of what is said. As we all know, often what we say is not exactly what we mean. When his mother sarcastically commented that Seth, who had ignored her request to clean his room, "was doing a really good job," he nodded and continued playing Nintendo. He didn't appreciate his mother's frustration, conveyed by her tone of voice and facial expression, or notice the mismatch between her statement and the context. Another boy, when I called his house and asked if his mother was home, answered "Yes" and then hung up the phone. He took my question literally, rather than understanding it as a polite but indirect way of asking to speak to his mother.

Still another common communication problem of people with AS-HFA is *how* they speak. Children with these disorders may speak very loudly or, conversely, too softly to be heard well. Words may tumble out of their mouths at breakneck speed or crawl out as if on a recording played at the wrong speed. Or their speech may have an unusual rhythm, with emphasis placed on the wrong words in sentences, a rising conclusion to a statement, making it sound like a question, or little inflection, giving their voice a flat tone. There may be fewer of the natural pauses we usually make in conversation, resulting in run-on speech. Or they may take breaths at unusual points during speaking, such as in the middle of a word or phrase. Often children with AS-HFA are unaware of how different from others they sound.

Unusual Interests and Behaviors

The third area in which people with high-functioning autism spectrum disorders differ is behavior. You will probably have noticed that your child's range of activities is relatively focused and that he or she can do the same thing over and over again without getting bored. Among those with Asperger syndrome and high-functioning autism, these traits usually show up as very specific interests that verge on obsessions. These kids have the favorite pastimes that many children have—computers, video games, dinosaurs, astronomy—but pursue them to the exclusion of almost everything else. Many parents report that their child will stay at the computer for hours, not breaking to go to the toilet, to eat, or to sleep unless pressured, and even then with much resistance. The intensity of the child's interests seems odd to others and may contribute to the child's social isolation. So does the child's choice of interests. Few "typical" children (or adults) appreciate the intricacies of the stock market, the seven deadly sins, sprinkler systems, or botanical classification, but these are the types of things that children with AS-HFA tend to favor. Their interests often revolve around topics about which the child can amass a great deal of facts and information. Sometimes these children also form unusual collections. One teenage girl with high-functioning autism saved the little sticker from every banana and apple she had ever eaten, keeping them in a treasured scrapbook that she carried with her everywhere.

What many onlookers find even more puzzling about children with Asperger syndrome or high-functioning autism is that, despite all the time they spend on these interests, the children often do not have good commonsense knowledge of their favorite subjects. They zero in on detail but are often unable to see "the big picture." One young man with high-functioning autism we saw in our research study for many years was very interested in vacuum cleaners. He knew everything there was to know about vacuums: the cost, color, repair record, and number and kinds of attachments for every brand on the market. He correctly identified my (S.O.) home vacuum as "tan with chocolate-brown trim" with two attachments, one hose-like and one with a brush. Its repair record was not good, he explained to me, since most of the internal parts were made of plastic rather than metal (in fact, it did not seem to work too well!). But when asked for advice about replacing it with a better one, the boy became agitated and eventually advised me to purchase a Royal, justifying this choice by explaining that it has a blue bag. Like many children with AS-HFA, he seemed unable to distinguish important details from irrelevant ones and to weigh the multiple details he had memorized. If your child has AS-HFA, you may notice that he or she has the same problem with thinking in general, demonstrating an excellent memory for facts but more difficulty understanding abstract concepts and using common sense. If you give your child a rule, he or she may have trouble generalizing it to a slightly different situation. Your child may want to solve problems the exact same way each time and may get very frustrated when you try to help him or her see new solutions or ways of doing things. The difficulty with seeing relationships among pieces of information, identifying central patterns or themes, and figuring out what things *mean* can make learning challenging for children with AS-HFA, as we discuss in Chapter 7.

The Strengths That Accompany the Challenges

Having Asperger syndrome or high-functioning autism is not all bad. There are special gifts, talents, and inclinations that come along with the challenges and make your child a very special, unique, and interesting person. Many children and teens with these conditions have excellent memories. They remember details of family trips, routes around their city, or spelling lists effortlessly. Many also excel in reading. Like Joseph, they may teach themselves to read at an early age and later be able to read words aloud and spell well above grade level. Others are very advanced in visual–spatial skills, putting together complex jigsaw puzzles, reading maps, or working electronic equipment far better than their peers. If you can find some practical way to apply your child's special interests to the "real world," then his or her incredible abilities to focus, memorize, and spend long hours immersed in a topic become invaluable strengths. You may have heard of Dr. Temple Grandin, a professor of animal science at Colorado State University, who has high-functioning autism. She combined a strong interest in animals with her visual–spatial strengths to revolutionize the design of animal slaughterhouses, making them more humane as well as more efficient. She has become an international expert on the topic, giving lectures around the world. For careers that rely on detail orientation, such as library administration, engineering, or computer science, having Asperger syndrome or high-functioning autism might be an asset. Your child thinks, views the world, processes information, and has a personality style that is different but not inferior. Great strengths come with the challenges. *Our* challenge is to harness those strengths and use them to overcome the hurdles that stand in the way. Chapter 5 offers practical suggestions for meeting that challenge.

What Lies Ahead?

The combination of challenges and talents seen in children with AS-HFA strikes fear in the hearts of many parents. Which will prevail, the child's deficiencies or the child's strengths? What can you do to make sure that your child doesn't slip through the cracks because his or her needs are not as extreme as those of children with more severe autism? What are your child's chances of going to college, getting a good job, and marrying? When a child displays such a mixture of challenges and strengths, it is often difficult to predict what the future holds. Of course, what may lie ahead is one of the first questions parents ask.

We see tremendous variability in individuals with AS-HFA as they get older. Some go to college, develop successful careers, and form lasting friendships, while others continue to live with family members and are underemployed in jobs that do not take advantage of their intelligence and special abilities. Adults with AS-HFA, such as Temple Grandin and Liane Willey, have written books that eloquently describe overcoming early challenges and successfully adapting to society (see the Appendix). In contrast, most research studies find a variety of residual social difficulties and low rates of independent living and full-time, unsupported employment even in very high-functioning adults.

Our ability to predict the future for children with AS-HFA is still limited. While we are beginning to understand the wide range of possibilities, we don't yet know how to match specific early characteristics with later outcomes. Research is not as helpful as we might hope, because the study participants were either diagnosed with more classic autism in childhood or were diagnosed late in life (since the field did not generally appreciate the existence of AS-HFA until recently) and therefore did not receive the treatments that we now believe are very helpful. Dr. Kanner predicted that the outcome for people with autism might improve in the future as the disorder became better recognized and new treatments were developed—just as we've seen with bipolar disorder and other disorders that once came with a poor prognosis. Recent studies have in fact found that very poor outcomes, such as institutionalization, are rare nowadays. As individuals with AS-HFA are diagnosed earlier and provided with state-of-the-art treatments, we expect that the rate of the best outcomes, including satisfying careers and independent living, will continue to increase. In this section, we briefly describe what is currently known about how AS-HFA unfolds and what might happen in adulthood. Much more on this topic appears in Chapter 9.

As with many conditions that begin in childhood, both the challenges and the triumphs of AS-HFA change over the person's lifespan. Symptoms begin in infancy in most cases, increase for a few years, usually peak in the preschool period, and then begin to level off or decline in the school-age years. Virtually everyone with high-functioning autism or Asperger syndrome improves with time and age. Children learn to express themselves through language and understand language better as time goes on. They become more and more interested in social contact, and they gain skills such as making conversation and using eye contact appropriately. Still, most children will continue to qualify for a diagnosis of AS-HFA as teenagers and adults. In a recent study by Dr. Joseph Piven, a child psychiatrist at the University of North Carolina at Chapel Hill, 82% of the high-functioning adolescents and adults with autism spectrum disorders they worked with had made significant improvements in social behavior and communication skills since childhood, but they all still met the criteria that define autism spectrum conditions. Many adults with high-functioning autism or Asperger syndrome admit they still feel somewhat awkward or unsure of themselves when talking to and interacting with others; their speech is still often very formal; and they still have trouble knowing how much to say or when to stop talking. In all the studies conducted so far, good verbal ability and average or better intelligence in childhood seemed to be the keys to predicting a good outcome in adulthood. This means that the children of most of you reading this book will have relatively good outcomes, at least compared to children with more severe autism, who have both lower verbal ability and lower intelligence than your child. There is reason for hope.

As to how the future looks for children with Asperger syndrome compared to those with high-functioning autism, we have only a few studies that have compared the two. A Swedish study conducted in 1997 found that adults with Asperger syndrome were more likely to have been in mainstream school and to have married than those with high-functioning autism; however, the groups did not differ in the number attending college or holding jobs. It's hard to know if the differences found between the conditions are due to their diagnoses or their intelligence, however, since the group with Asperger syndrome in this particular study was brighter, on average, than the group with high-functioning autism. As part of a long-term study being conducted in my laboratory in Salt Lake City, we found that adolescents with Asperger syndrome had more years of regular education, better expressive language, and more highly developed imagination and creativity than those with high-functioning autism and the same intelligence level. But to conclude that the future looks brighter for those with Asperger syndrome than for those with high-functioning autism would be premature. We still are not completely certain how to differentiate the two disorders—more on this in Chapter 2—so making any definitive statements about the differences between the two would be premature. Dr. Patricia Howlin, a psychologist in Great Britain who has written a great deal about outcome in adult life for individuals with AS-HFA, concludes that while some individuals may succeed as adults, such achievements rarely come easily and may depend just as much on the available support systems (parents, intervention programs, educational accommodations) as on the individual's personal characteristics and abilities. She describes how the pressure to fit into a culture with very different values can come at a high cost, including stress, anxiety, and depression. Even when adults with AS-HFA achieve important milestones, like graduating from college and establishing careers, they may struggle with independent living. Seth's mother summarized both her hopes and her fears by saying, "I bet he'll become a rocket scientist, but I'll probably have to dress him and drive him to work."

Are You and Your Child Alone in This?

As you search for answers about how and why your child is so different, you may feel tremendously alone. You may have spent years feeling that no one else has a child just like yours. In fact you may never have heard of high-functioning autism or Asperger syndrome before your doctor or someone else raised it. Actually, you're not nearly as alone as you may now feel. Prevalence estimates vary widely, with numbers as high as 1% of the school-age population occasionally suggested for the whole autism spectrum and between 0.2 and 0.5% (or 2 to 5 individuals in 1,000) with Asperger syndrome alone. Many researchers believe these numbers are high, but even more conservative estimates suggest that autism spectrum disorders are much more common than we initially thought. As recently as 10–15 years ago, we estimated only 2–4 of every 10,000 individuals had an autism-related condition. But a very recent (2001) study published in the prestigious *Journal of the American Medical Association* found a much higher rate. The research team of Dr. Eric Fombonne, a prominent French epidemiologist (a scientist who investigates the rate of diseases in the community), studied over 15,000 individuals in a region of England, identifying every case of autism spectrum disorders in the geographical area (verifying the diagnoses themselves). They found a rate of 63 people with autism spectrum disorders in every 10,000 individuals in the general population, making autism spectrum disorders more common than Down syndrome and many other childhood conditions. Only about a quarter of the individuals with autism spectrum disorders in this epidemiological study were diagnosed with classic autism. Fully three-quarters of the children had diagnoses in the high-functioning end of the autism spectrum. This suggests that children like yours are actually more common than "typical" children with autism.

If we now think that autism spectrum disorders are 15–30 times more common than we did a decade ago, a question naturally arises: Is autism increasing in frequency? Is it truly more common than it used to be, or do the rising prevalence figures simply reflect better diagnostic practices and increased awareness of the milder end of the continuum? The jury is still out. Two researchers, Dr. Lorna Wing (the same psychiatrist who first brought Asperger syndrome to the attention of the English-speaking world) and Dr. Eric Fombonne, the French epidemiologist, recently reviewed all studies of the prevalence of autism spectrum disorders ever conducted. Independently, both concluded that there is no evidence that autism is increasing in frequency; both suggested that the apparent increase comes from the fact that children with AS-HFA symptoms are more likely to be referred to a professional who can diagnose them accurately and from the fact that the criteria used to diagnose AS-HFA have been fine-tuned. Professionals are now better at diagnosing individuals with autism spectrum disorders, especially high-functioning ones, as well as more willing to make such diagnoses, as better community services become available. Some scientists still suspect that environmental factors increase the risk for autism and account for increased prevalence rates, however. This is an active area of investigation at research centers around the world.

Another factor that may influence prevalence estimates is the rate of misdiagnosis. As the label of Asperger syndrome has become better known by professionals, both its use and its misuse have increased. Every day, many children with multiple, difficult, complex developmental and behavioral problems are seen in clinics around the world, and the professionals who see them can occasionally be at a loss for a diagnosis. With the advent of the "Asperger" label, some of these children have been diagnosed with Asperger syndrome. Some indeed have it, but many do not, as we discuss in more detail in Chapter 2. A similar phenomenon occurred a decade ago with attention-deficit/hyperactivity disorder (ADHD), which some observers now consider overdiagnosed or applied inappropriately. Such developments are usually guided by a desire to advocate for children and help them obtain services, but in the process they exaggerate the prevalence of the disorders. If high-functioning autism spectrum disorders become the ADHD of the new millennium, we will certainly see prevalence estimates increasing, although not necessarily due to an actual increase in the frequency of the disorder.

All autism spectrum disorders are much more common in males than in females; this was recognized by both Leo Kanner and Hans Asperger and has been validated by numerous studies since then. Four boys are diagnosed with classic autism for every one girl with the disorder. The male-to-female ratio is even wider for high-functioning forms, such as Asperger syndrome and high-functioning autism. Some researchers have found 10 boys with these milder conditions for each affected girl. This lower risk may be good news for parents of baby girls, particularly those who follow an older brother with autism. In fact, boys are at greater risk than girls for virtually all developmental, behavioral, and learning disorders. However, the data also mean that girls with autism spectrum disorders seem less likely than boys to have a high-functioning form of the disorder.

The reason that girls are affected less often than boys is not yet clear. As you will read in Chapter 3, autism spectrum disorders seem to have multiple causes, and more than one factor may have to be present for the disorder to develop. It has been speculated that there is something about being a girl (perhaps a different prenatal hormonal environment or sex-related patterns of brain organization) that "protects" females from autism and other developmental problems. With such protective factors present, the risk for developing disorders is lower in girls than boys and may require the presence of more of these causative factors. Then, with multiple problems affecting their brains, girls end up being relatively more severely affected, on the average. This hypothesis is speculative, but research teams are currently studying such possibilities.

In this first chapter, we described the high-functioning autism spectrum disorders and how they influence the lives of affected children and their families. Our goal, at this point, is to help you decide whether the diagnoses of Asperger syndrome and high-functioning autism are relevant to the person in your life you are worried about and whether this book will help you in your search for answers. The next chapter will explain how professionals currently arrive at diagnoses of high-functioning autism and Asperger syndrome and which conditions can be confused with AS-HFA. The more you know about the diagnostic process, the greater power you have to ensure that your child receives the most accurate diagnosis possible.

CHAPTER 2

The Diagnostic Process

After hearing the school psychologist's concerns about Asperger syndrome, Lauren's parents began reading everything they could get their hands on about the condition. The label seemed to fit Lauren well in some ways, particularly her lack of friends and trouble looking people in the eye, but other features, like overly formal language and clumsiness, just didn't sound like their daughter. The school psychologist felt pretty strongly that a diagnosis of Asperger syndrome explained Lauren's challenges and would help her obtain needed services but suggested they get a second opinion, recommending a child psychiatrist in town with experience in autism spectrum disorders. At the request of the psychiatrist, Lauren's parents obtained copies of her medical records from their pediatrician. In a report dictated after Lauren's 3-year check-up, they read, "This young girl, born prematurely, is now thriving. She is physically well developed, alert, and happy, although she is described by her parents as quite shy and fearful. We spent some time assessing development. She played alone throughout the visit and rarely looked up at the adults. She was having difficulty focusing on tasks. . . . Lauren clearly has some interaction difficulties, though her relatedness is probably okay for age." Lauren's parents were startled that the doctor had noted, way back then, their daughter's solitariness, and were both confused and frustrated by the conclusion. Why hadn't this been figured out sooner?

At age 2, Seth was not yet talking and seemed indifferent to his siblings and parents. When people called his name or spoke to him, he didn't appear to hear them. His parents were sure he wasn't deaf, as he would perk up whenever the automatic garage door opened, even when he was in distant parts of the house. But just to be on the safe side, Seth's parents had his hearing tested. The results were perfectly normal, but the audiologist asked them if they had ever considered autism. This diagnosis was confirmed by a child psychologist at age 3. Seth was immediately enrolled in a special education preschool for children with autism. He began talking quickly and made rapid progress in all areas, such that he was able to enter kindergarten in a regular classroom with just some minimal assistance from an aide. As he began school, his parents were told that he did not have autism, but actually something called Asperger syndrome. Who was right?

There are many routes through the maze of diagnosis, some direct, others taking trips down blind alleys and leading to dead ends. In this chapter, we help you find your way by explaining the specific diagnostic criteria for Asperger syndrome, high-functioning autism, and related disorders, including similarities and differences. We'll tell you how a diagnostic evaluation is conducted and how diagnostic decisions about your child should be made; we will also discuss conditions sometimes confused with autism spectrum disorders.

The Diagnostic Bible: DSM-IV

The diagnostic process varies from agency to agency and from professional to professional. Some evaluations are comprehensive and lengthy, others relatively quick. Some professionals will use special tests, while others will talk with you and play with your child in a seemingly informal manner. But all will be collecting specific information about your child's early development and current strengths and weaknesses in the three areas relevant to autism spectrum disorders. As we outlined in Chapter 1, these areas are your child's social interaction skills, ability to communicate with others, and special interests or unusual behaviors. Once this information is collected, a decision is made about whether your child meets criteria for an autism spectrum disorder and, if so, which one. To do this, professionals use the American Psychiatric Association's *Diagnostic and Statistical Manual of Mental Disorders* (or DSM), which outlines the specific behaviors and problems associated with each condition. The DSM is currently in its fourth edition, known as the DSM-IV (pronounced "DSM-four"). The DSM is revised every 5 to 10 years to reflect new knowledge amassed by clinicians and researchers in mental health. If your child was diagnosed some time ago, then an earlier edition may have been used, probably either the DSM-III (the third edition) or the DSM-III-R (the revised third edition). If you live outside the United States, the manual called the *International Classification of Diseases* (or ICD), may have been used instead. Asperger syndrome was first included in these diagnostic manuals in the 1990s, so only individuals evaluated in the last few years will have been given this diagnosis.

The DSM-IV helps mental health professionals diagnose all emotional, behavioral, and mental conditions, including depression, anxiety, hyperactivity, and schizophrenia. All specific diagnoses are included within categories—for example, depression falls within the "Mood Disorders" category, while phobias fall under the "Anxiety Disorders" category. The category that contains the autism spectrum disorders is called "Pervasive Developmental Disorders."[1] This umbrella term was used by the authors of the DSM to differentiate autism spectrum conditions from more specific developmental disorders, like learning disabilities. Children with pervasive developmental disorders, including Asperger syndrome and high-functioning autism, experience difficulty across multiple (or "pervasive") areas of development (social, communication, behavior, cognition, sometimes even motor skills). In contrast, children with specific developmental disorders, like dyslexia, have problems in only one specific learning area (such as reading), but function okay in other subjects, are quite normal socially and behaviorally, and have at least average motor skills.

There are five specific conditions within the Pervasive Developmental Disorder, or PDD, category: autistic disorder, Asperger disorder,[2] Rett's disorder, childhood disintegrative disorder, and pervasive developmental disorder not otherwise specified (PDDNOS). The five

----

[1]The term *Pervasive Developmental Disorders* can be considered synonymous with autism spectrum disorders.

[2]The DSM uses the more technical labels "Asperger disorder" and "autistic disorder," rather than the terms Asperger syndrome and autism you may be used to. There are no differences between these terms and they can be considered synonyms. In other words, it doesn't matter if your doctor tells you that your child has Asperger syndrome or Asperger disorder; they are the same thing.

disorders differ from one another in specific ways, but equally important is what they all share. First, each of the five PDD conditions involves *pervasive* difficulties across multiple areas of development. Second, each involves significant impairment in relating socially to others. Although individuals with other disabilities, such as mental retardation (without autism), have pervasive difficulties across multiple domains, such individuals do not exhibit significant social impairment. Rather, their social abilities are commensurate with their mental abilities. In contrast, the social impairment of individuals with PDD often is more severe than what one would expect for their mental abilities.

Two of the conditions in the autism spectrum, namely Rett's disorder and childhood disintegrative disorder, are almost always associated with significant cognitive impairment and are not considered among the high-functioning autism spectrum disorders. These two conditions are briefly described below.

Rett's Disorder

Children with both Rett's disorder and childhood disintegrative disorder have very severe impairments in thinking and learning skills, in addition to their social, communication, and behavioral problems. Both conditions involve a period of normal development followed by a loss of skills. Rett's disorder is found only in girls. The baby appears fine at birth and develops normally for at least 5 months (and often longer), attaining head control, following objects and people with her eyes, rolling over, and sitting by herself. But within 6 months to a year or two later, she begins to lose interest in others and in social interaction. The growth of her head slows down, probably reflecting slowing in brain development. Depending on how old she is when the regression begins, the little girl with Rett's disorder may lose specific speech, thinking, and motor skills; if she is young, then her development in these areas plateaus, without her attaining the skills parents expect (pointing, playing with toys, walking, talking, and so on). One of the most difficult problems faced by girls with Rett's disorder is very poor use of their hands. Instead of using them to play, handle things, or explore their world, they repetitively wring, "wash," twist, clap, or rub their hands together in the middle of their body. This is a nearly constant behavior that obviously interferes with the little girl's ability to do almost everything. Girls with Rett's disorder are much more severely limited in their development than children with higher-functioning autism spectrum disorders like Asperger syndrome and mild autism.

Childhood Disintegrative Disorder

Like Rett's disorder, childhood disintegrative disorder involves a period of normal development followed by a loss of skills, resulting in severe impairments in cognitive, self-help, and other skills. The pattern is somewhat different from Rett's, however, and the two are easily distinguished. Childhood disintegrative disorder can occur in either boys or girls but is much more common in boys. The hand movements so typical of Rett's are not seen in childhood disintegrative disorder. Also, the period of normal development is longer than in Rett's: the regression occurs after at least 2 (and up to 10) years of normal development. Prior to the regression, the child appears perfectly normal, interacting with others, talking, playing, and taking care of him- or herself at the level appropriate for his or her age (for example, using the toilet and eating independently). There is then a loss of skills, with the child withdrawing, no longer talking, losing thinking skills, bowel control, and other abilities. Both Rett's and childhood disintegrative disorder are much less common than the other autism spectrum disorders. Note that if the child's loss of skills, often referred to as autistic regression, occurs before the age of 2 years, a diagnosis of autism rather than childhood disintegrative disorder is given. Currently, we do not understand why some children with PDD have symptoms from early infancy whereas others do not develop symptoms until later in life. This is an active area of research.

High-Functioning Autism

A child who is diagnosed with autistic disorder, the formal name given to autism in the DSM-IV, has difficulties in three areas: social relating, communication, and behaviors and interests. In Table 1, we've listed the specific behaviors (or symptoms) of autism described in the DSM-IV. More detailed descriptions of these behaviors are provided in Chapter 1. To meet DSM-IV criteria for autism, your child must display at

Table 1. DSM–IV Criteria for Autistic Disorder

DSM-IV symptoms	Examples

Deficits in reciprocal social interaction

DSM-IV symptoms	Examples
1a. Difficulty using nonverbal behaviors to regulate social interaction	• Trouble looking others in the eye • Little use of gestures while speaking • Few or unusual facial expressions • Trouble knowing how close to stand to others • Unusual intonation or voice quality
1b. Failure to develop age-appropriate peer relationships	• Few or no friends • Relationships only with those much older or younger than the child or with family members • Relationships based primarily on special interests • Trouble interacting in groups and following cooperative rules of games
1c. Little sharing of pleasure, achievements, or interests with others	• Enjoys favorite activities, television shows, toys alone, without trying to involve other people • Does not try to call others' attention to activities, interests, or accomplishments • Little interest in or reaction to praise
1d. Lack of social or emotional reciprocity	• Does not respond to others; "appears deaf" • Not aware of others; "oblivious" to their existence • Strongly prefers solitary activities • Does not notice when others are hurt or upset; does not offer comfort

Deficits in communication

DSM-IV symptoms	Examples
2a. Delay in or total lack of development of language	• No use of words to communicate by age 2 • No simple phrases (for example, "More milk") by age 3 • After speech develops, immature grammar or repeated errors
2b. Difficulty holding conversations	• Has trouble knowing how to start, keep going, and/or end a conversation • Little back-and-forth; may talk on and on in a monologue • Fails to respond to the comments of others; responds only to direct questions • Difficulty talking about topics not of special interest
2c. Unusual or repetitive language	• Repeating what others say to them (echolalia) • Repeating from videos, books, or commercials at inappropriate times or out of context • Using words or phrases that the child has made up or that have special meaning only to him/her • Overly formal, pedantic style of speaking (sounds like "a little professor")

(cont.)

Table 1 (cont.)

DSM-IV symptoms	Examples
2d. Play that is not appropriate for developmental level	• Little acting-out scenarios with toys • Rarely pretends an object is something else (for example, a banana is a telephone) • Prefers to use toys in a concrete manner (for example, building with blocks, arranging dollhouse furniture) rather than pretending with them • When young, little interest in social games like peekaboo, ring-around-the-rosie, and the like

Restricted, repetitive behaviors, interests or activities

3a. Interests that are narrow in focus, overly intense, and/or unusual	• Very strong focus on particular topics to the exclusion of other topics • Difficulty "letting go" of special topics or activities • Interference with other activities (for example, delays eating or toileting due to focus on activity) • Interest in topics that are unusual for age (sprinkler systems, movie ratings, astrophysics, radio station call letters) • Excellent memory for details of special interests
3b. Unreasonable insistence on sameness and following familiar routines	• Wants to perform certain activities in an exact order (for example, close car doors in specific order) • Easily upset by minor changes in routine (for example, taking a different route home from school) • Need for advanced warning of any changes • Becomes highly anxious and upset if routines or rituals not followed
3c. Repetitive motor mannerisms	• Flapping hands when excited or upset • Flicking fingers in front of eyes • Odd hand postures or other hand movements • Spinning or rocking for long periods of time • Walking and/or running on tiptoe
3d. Preoccupation with parts of objects	• Uses objects in unusual ways (for example, flicks doll's eyes, repeatedly opens and closes doors on toy car), rather than as intended • Interest in sensory qualities of objects (for example, likes to sniff objects or look at them closely) • Likes objects that move (for example, fans, running water, spinning wheels) • Attachment to unusual objects (orange peel, string)

least six of the 12 symptoms listed. Your child may meet criteria for a specific symptom if he or she displays one or more of the behaviors associated with that symptom (listed in the right-hand column of Table 1).[3] Children diagnosed with autism must experience at least two of the symptoms in the "reciprocal social interaction" domain, at least one symptom in the "communication" domain, and at least one symptom in the "restricted, repetitive behaviors" domain. At least one difficulty must have been present before age 3. If your child fulfills these criteria (number of symptoms, pattern of symptoms across the three domains, and age of onset), then he or she will be diagnosed with autistic disorder.

What about high-functioning autism? This is the term used for children who meet autistic disorder criteria but have relatively normal thinking and learning skills (that is, they are not mentally retarded) and language skills (they can speak close to the level expected for their age). At least a quarter to a third of children diagnosed with autistic disorder fall within this special subgroup that we call "high-functioning autism," although recent studies suggest the proportion may be even higher.

Not everyone diagnosed with autism displays every symptom listed in Table 1. Only six symptoms are required, and there is no particular behavior or problem that everyone diagnosed with autism must show. This means that you may read accounts of autism that do not sound like your child. You may know a neighborhood boy with autism who seems quite different from your son. You may have heard that all children with autism are unaffectionate, but your child loves hugs, kisses, and cuddles on your lap. Thus it is likely that some things about the diagnosis fit your child while others do not, as Lauren's parents experienced; this does not necessarily indicate that your child was diagnosed incorrectly.

Asperger Syndrome

Now to Asperger syndrome. Its symptoms are identical to those listed in Table 1 for autistic disorder, except that there is no requirement that the child demonstrate significant difficulties in the second category:

---

[3]But, of course, determination of which specific symptoms are present must be made by a doctor with appropriate training.

communication. In other words, individuals with Asperger syndrome have the same types of reciprocal social interaction deficits and re-stricted, repetitive behaviors as individuals with autism but don't dis-play the same language difficulties. No matter how old they are, their language ability is about what would be expected for their age, espe-cially in the areas of grammar, vocabulary, or pronunciation. It is, in fact, a specific requirement of the Asperger diagnosis that language de-velop at the normal time, with the child saying words by age 2 and us-ing simple phrases ("Go bye-bye," "My ball") by age 3. Sometimes lan-guage may even be precocious in its development. Some of the children described by Dr. Asperger talked before they walked. Many, like Jo-seph, completely bypass baby talk, sounding like adults when they are only 2 or 3 years old. A second criterion for the Asperger diagnosis, be-yond normal language development, is normal intelligence. This is gen-erally defined as an IQ score above 70 on a test of intelligence (more on this in the section on testing). Because of their good language and cog-nitive skills, the parents of children with Asperger syndrome may not be worried until their child enters school, when their social awkward-ness and obsessive interests become more obvious in comparison to other children.

Ever since Dr. Lorna Wing brought Asperger syndrome to the attention of the English-speaking world in the 1980s, researchers have been fascinated by its similarities to and differences from high-functioning autism. In terms of learning and thinking, different strengths and weaknesses may be associated with the two conditions. Dr. Leo Kanner, who first described autism, wrote about children with unusually strong visual–spatial abilities. For example, one boy de-scribed in Dr. Kanner's paper could complete puzzles "guided by form entirely, to the extent that it made no difference whether the pieces were right side up or not." Dr. Asperger, on the other hand, made no mention of special visual–spatial strengths, but did highlight the imagi-native, abstract, perspective-taking abilities of his patients. In his first paper describing the syndrome, he wrote: "Their thoughts can be un-usually rich. . . . One young boy surprised us with remarks that be-trayed an excellent apprehension of a situation and an accurate judg-ment of people. This was the more amazing as he apparently never took any notice of his environment." Dr. Asperger also wrote that his patients "know who means well with them and who does not." Some studies suggest that the ability to understand other people's intentions and perspectives may be better in people with Asperger syndrome than in those with autism.

While people with Asperger syndrome may, on the average, have better developed language, imagination, and perspective taking than those with high-functioning autism (and we are not entirely sure this is true; our understanding of the syndrome is still growing), they are not less impaired in all areas. Dr. Asperger noticed that all his patients were very clumsy and often were late to walk and develop other motor skills. Most were poor at sports and strongly disliked physical education classes at school. Dr. Asperger described their handwriting as "atrocious." Some recent research has indeed found that children with Asperger syndrome are clumsier than those with high-functioning autism, but other studies have not. For now, the jury is out and more research is needed.

A second area in which the two conditions may differ is in the nature of their repetitive behaviors. Some researchers have found that children with Asperger syndrome are more likely to have obsessive interests in narrow or unusual topics (such as Joseph's fascination with geography), while children with autism (high-functioning as well as more severe autism) are more likely to display repetitive hand mannerisms or to use objects in unusual ways (see Table 1). As with the research on clumsiness, however, the results of these studies are not consistent and we don't yet know for sure if this pattern really does distinguish one condition from the other.

Distinguishing High-Functioning Autism from Asperger Syndrome: Is There a Difference?

The characteristics that may differentiate autism from Asperger syndrome are so tentative that they have not been included in the DSM-IV. There is, for example, no requirement in the DSM-IV that children with Asperger syndrome must be clumsy to meet criteria for the diagnosis. Likewise, there is nothing that says that everyone with autism must be good at puzzles (or that those with Asperger syndrome must be poor at puzzles). So how do we distinguish between the two? Unfortunately, it's a very common experience for parents to receive different opinions, with one professional diagnosing Asperger syndrome and another telling you that it is actually high-functioning autism. Right now, the only reliable way to tell which condition your child has is to rule out the diagnosis of Asperger syndrome if he or she meets the criteria for autism. In the DSM-IV, the autism diagnosis always takes precedence over the Asperger syndrome diagnosis. This means that if your child meets autism criteria (showing at least six symptoms from Table 1, with at least two in the social domain, one in the communication domain, and one in the repetitive behavior area, and at least one symptom was present by age 3), then he or she is diagnosed with autism, regardless of whether the Asperger diagnosis also seems to fit. Another way to look at this is that children who are correctly diagnosed with Asperger syndrome fail to meet the autism criteria in some way. Perhaps they didn't show any difficulties before age 3 or maybe they don't have any symptoms in the communication domain or possibly they do not display the minimum of six symptoms required for a DSM-IV diagnosis of autism.[4]

Okay, you may say, my son does seem to meet autism criteria by those rules, *but* he talked very early and always had an advanced vocabulary, like Joseph. Interestingly, research by scientists in both the United States and Australia shows that some children with high-functioning autism do indeed talk at the normal time. Talking on time is not enough to qualify for a diagnosis of Asperger syndrome; the child must have talked on time *and* failed to meet autism criteria.

As you may have figured out at this point, the distinction between high-functioning autism and Asperger syndrome can be made only by counting symptoms and asking specific questions about language development at ages 2 and 3. Most professionals would agree that these are small differences. Observing a group of children, some of whom were diagnosed with Asperger syndrome and others of whom were diagnosed with high-functioning autism, both parents and professionals alike would be hard-pressed to know which child had which condition. The practical significance of the difference may be minor. Does it matter if your child's language was a bit delayed at age 2, as long as he

....

[4]In our experience, the majority of children with Asperger syndrome fail to meet autism criteria for the third reason, namely, that they display fewer than six symptoms from Table 1.

speaks fine now? The fact of the matter is that he needs the same treatment as the child who talked fine at age 2, but who shares your child's difficulties in looking people in the eye and making friends. That is why we devote this book to both conditions.

PDDNOS

The fifth and final condition that falls within the PDD category is pervasive developmental disorder not otherwise specified (or PDDNOS). This label is used for children who have clear difficulty relating to others, as well as either communication problems or repetitive behaviors, but who do not meet criteria for any of the other PDDs. The same list of symptoms outlined in Table 1 is used to diagnose PDDNOS, but these children must demonstrate only one difficulty within the "reciprocal social interaction" domain and one symptom from either the "communication deficits" or "repetitive, restricted behaviors" domains. Although they have autistic-like behaviors and difficulties, they do not meet the full criteria for either autism or Asperger syndrome. Usually they have either too few symptoms or the wrong pattern of symptoms.

Chad has difficulty looking people in the eye, dislikes changes in routine, and checks Internet auction sites daily to bid on the action figures he collects. However, he doesn't show any other clear symptoms of autism spectrum disorders. He has several close friends, chats with others in a typical way, is highly imaginative, and his voice doesn't sound any different from other 9-year-old boys.

Chad is diagnosed with PDDNOS because he clearly has some difficulties associated with the autism spectrum but doesn't demonstrate either the number or pattern of symptoms required for diagnoses of high-functioning autism or Asperger syndrome. These conditions require at least two deficits in reciprocal social interaction, but Chad shows only one (difficulty with eye contact). He also demonstrates a total of only three symptoms, while at least six are required for an autism diagnosis.

Some professionals dislike the PDDNOS category because it is so mixed. Children whose symptoms fall within the category can be vastly different from each other. After all, only two symptoms from the list of 12 are needed for a diagnosis of PDDNOS, meaning that the number of possible symptom combinations is huge. Another problem with the PDDNOS label is that it is often misused. When research was being done to examine how well the third edition of the DSM worked and to make needed changes for the fourth edition, scientists found that many children with PDDNOS had been misdiagnosed. About a third of them actually met the full criteria for autism and thus would have been more appropriately diagnosed with high-functioning autism. And many others did not have any symptoms on the autism spectrum! This study found that most of the children labeled with PDDNOS who didn't have any specific symptoms related to autism or Asperger syndrome fell into two categories: those with general language or learning problems and mildly delayed social skills and those with hyperactive, distractible, highly disorganized behavior. In both cases, clinicians felt that other diagnoses (for example, mental retardation, ADHD) underestimated the severity and pervasiveness of the disturbance, so they diagnosed the child with PDDNOS even though the child did not actually meet diagnostic criteria. For this reason, many professionals will take a second look at any child diagnosed with PDDNOS to make sure that it is an accurate label. Certainly some children do meet the criteria for it, but it is clearly overdiagnosed.

Others defend the PDDNOS category, reasoning that there is a need to classify children who are legitimately experiencing problems, but who do not fit neatly into one category or another. Without a diagnosis, they would fall through the cracks of the system even more, perhaps not obtaining needed services or being labeled as disobedient, willful, or difficult, because no one appreciated the nature of their problems. Whether we like it or not, the specific conditions listed in the DSM, such as autism or Asperger syndrome, do not cover all possible variations of symptoms that appear in children. In fact, the DSM acknowledges this truth by including a "Not Otherwise Specified" (NOS) diagnosis within every type of disorder (for example, someone might be diagnosed with mood disorder NOS when he shows some symptoms of depression but does not meet full criteria for the disorder). In general, all NOS diagnoses in the DSM are reserved for those whose symptoms are atypical or fall below the threshold for other diagnoses but who are experiencing significant impairment and distress.

When PDDNOS is diagnosed accurately, it clearly falls on the autism spectrum. The problems experienced by children with PDDNOS cannot be explained by any other category of disorder. Children with learning disabilities, attention problems, or obsessive–compulsive disorder (OCD), for example, do not have the highly focused interests or trouble making eye contact that Chad has. Thus PDDNOS is best thought of as "atypical autism" (in fact, that is what European doctors call it). It involves autistic-type symptoms but is less severe and has a pattern of symptoms that is not quite the same as the patterns associated with high-functioning autism or Asperger syndrome. Yet the interventions that help children with these conditions also help those with PDDNOS, so this book will be helpful to parents of children with PDDNOS as well.

Is the Diagnosis Accurate?

After reading the last few pages, you may wonder what the odds are that your child will be (or has been) diagnosed accurately. Or you may actually have gotten two different labels for your child's difficulties, as Seth's mother did, and want to know how to find out which one is right. Or perhaps you think the diagnosis you've gotten exaggerates or minimizes your child's problem. What do you do? When parents do not feel confident in the diagnosis their child has received, it is sometimes helpful to get a second or even a third opinion until what you're told makes sense in the context of how well you know your child and what you know about PDDs. This is unfortunately a time-consuming and expensive process that many parents cannot afford. The following are our best, concise answers to questions that parents commonly raise about PDDs diagnoses.

How Can Different Evaluators Arrive at Different Diagnoses?

This is a very common occurrence (although no less frustrating because it is common). It comes about because professionals vary as to how strictly they adhere to the diagnostic "rules" outlined in the DSM-IV. Psychologists and psychiatrists who conduct research on autism spectrum disorders usually go by the book most carefully, as the seemingly minor differences between high-functioning autism and Asperger syndrome may be important to their investigations. Other professionals use the DSM criteria a bit more loosely. For example, some professionals diagnose any child with autistic-like behaviors who developed language by age 2 with Asperger syndrome, regardless of whether the other criteria for the disorder are met. Others steer away from the Asperger and PDDNOS labels, fearing they are less familiar to parents, the educational system, and insurance companies, possibly negatively affecting the services, resources, and benefits the child will be offered. One mother vented her frustrations by saying, "Try finding information on PDDNOS in a library or bookstore. I spent months looking until someone at my son's school told me that PDDNOS was related to autism." Therefore, some professionals may give all children with mild autism spectrum symptoms a diagnosis of high-functioning autism, regardless of the specific diagnostic criteria. Still other clinicians use the PDDNOS label liberally, even when the child meets autism criteria, because they feel that parents will find this label more reassuring than "autism." Some professionals might say that your child had autism when he was young but now has Asperger syndrome (even though the DSM does not allow children to "grow" from one diagnosis into another). Usually, such liberties with the diagnostic criteria are taken with the best of intentions, for example, to advocate for the child or to soften the blow for worried parents. And usually, these liberties have little practical significance. As long as you understand that all three conditions are highly related to each other and involve serious difficulties that require specific treatments, then it may not matter which of the three diagnoses your child received. The important point is that you know that all are *autism spectrum* conditions, and that services and resources for any one of the disorders are relevant and applicable to children with all three diagnoses.

What If One Professional Says My Child Has a PDD and Another Says He's Normal?

As we have emphasized throughout the first two chapters of this book, autistic-like behavior falls on a continuum. How often symptoms occur, how severe they are, how pervasive they are across different settings, how much they interfere with functioning, and how much distress they cause all factor into where your child falls on the spectrum and how close to what is considered "normal" he or she is. It's important to distinguish a diagnosis of AS-HFA from the little quirks and eccentricities that we all have. Most (but probably not all) symptoms of AS-HFA can be present in individuals without AS-HFA, but usually in much milder form. You may well know someone who is obsessed with a topic—say, model trains or computers—but who in other ways seems perfectly typical and not at all autistic. A neighbor of mine (S.O.), who is absolutely normal in all other ways, checks the Weather Channel on cable television a dozen times a day. He also enjoys keeping a list of when the sun rose and set in several cities around the world (usually places he and his wife have visited in their travels). Unlike people with AS-HFA, however, he does not tell others about this interest and in fact was a bit embarrassed when I happened upon the list as I was looking for a pen at his house one day. Or you may know someone who seems at a loss for words and appears quite anxious in social situations. Or you may have acquaintances who ramble on in excruciating detail and never seem to get to the point. Or you may know people who are quite orderly and become anxious when plans change. A colleague of ours, who is a very friendly and social woman, must plan her entire day in advance. If someone calls an unplanned meeting or invites her to lunch on the spur of the moment, she becomes quite unsettled, refuses the change when possible, and otherwise complains heartily of the disruption in her day. Any of these folks could have AS-HFA if, in addition to the one oddity described, they demonstrated other characteristic symptoms of AS-HFA. However, each of these oddities, when they occur in isolation and in the context of otherwise normal social relating and communication, are simply normal personality variants. What this means is that much of AS-HFA is on a continuum with "normal" (we won't get into the debate about what "normal" actually means here). The behaviors of people with AS-HFA are something that the rest of the non-AS-HFA world might at times experience or that might feel "normal" to them. The difference, however, between someone who has AS-HFA and someone who does not is the severity of the disturbance, in terms of both the number of "odd" or autistic-like behaviors and how much these quirks interfere with functioning and daily living.

How Can We Be Sure Our Child Has AS-HFA and Not ADHD . . . or OCD . . . or Something Else?

Estimates of the prevalence of autism spectrum disorders have soared during the past two decades. Although it is still unclear what has caused this rapid rise, one factor that has certainly contributed is that as professionals and the general public have become more familiar with the autism spectrum disorders, the number of children diagnosed with them has soared. And as their diagnosis has become more prevalent, misdiagnosis is also more likely. Sometimes a proper assessment by a specialist reveals that this diagnosis is wrong. It's been our experience that in earlier years almost all children referred to our specialty clinics for a diagnostic evaluation did in fact meet criteria for an autism spectrum disorder. In the last year alone, however, one-quarter of the diagnostic evaluations performed in our clinics overturned previously suggested diagnoses of either high-functioning autism or Asperger syndrome.[5] Almost all the children had multiple serious behavioral difficulties. It was never a straightforward case of dyslexia or ADHD having been misdiagnosed as Asperger syndrome, but one of a child presenting a complicated picture made up of many serious difficulties. During training, most professionals, regardless of specialty, are encouraged to use the fewest diagnoses possible for one individual. When reasonable, we try to summarize difficulties under one diagnosis rather than listing three or four separate conditions.[6] The term *pervasive developmental disorders* emphasizes that the difficulties experienced by the person are widespread and cut across several areas of development. If a clinician is not completely familiar with the specific diagnostic criteria, the diagnosis might appear to fit children with multiple complex difficulties, such as language delays, irritability, high activity level, and learning problems; there is no doubt that their problems are *pervasive*. But as you know from reading this chapter, the term *pervasive developmental disorders* is reserved for children with specific autistic-like difficulties, not any type of broad or general disability.

A second reason for misdiagnosis is that the symptoms of certain disorders do have some overlap, at least superficially, with the symptoms of AS-HFA. Obsessive–compulsive disorder (OCD) is a condition

---

[5]Rates of "delabeling" children are similar in other communities. A large center in Boston also reported that 15 to 25% of their clients did not meet criteria for the autism spectrum condition with which they had been previously diagnosed.

[6]This practice is sometimes referred to as the "law of parsimony" or "Occam's razor." William of Occam was an English philosopher of the early 14th century who stated that it should be a goal of science to first attempt to explain unknown phenomena in the simplest manner. The law of parsimony is exemplified in medical diagnostics by the saying, "When you hear hoofbeats, think horses, not zebras."

in which people have persistent thoughts or ideas that they have trouble getting out of their heads; they also feel extremely strong urges to perform certain behaviors or rituals. They often like to have things "just so" and become anxious or upset if things are not how they are used to or how they expect. Chris, a 12-year-old with OCD, had a favorite number (4) and felt compelled to perform actions and repeat certain phrases he had heard four times. If he didn't do this, he would become extremely nervous. The only way he could make his anxiety go away would be by making a quick sweeping motion on the floor with the back of his hand. Such unusual rituals may be somewhat reminiscent of the nonfunctional rituals of the autism spectrum (in Table 1, this is listed as symptom 3b). Take Mark, for example, a young boy with Asperger syndrome who screams and cries if his family doesn't shut the doors of the car and fasten their seatbelts in a clockwise order. He is insistent that everyone get out of the car and repeat the process in the "right" order—and his family is willing to do this to avoid Mark's serious distress that otherwise results. Mark's rituals don't make any sense to others and don't seem to be functional in any way, just like Chris's rituals. Both boys experience tremendous anxiety when things aren't done just the way they want. Yet one boy is diagnosed with OCD and the other with Asperger syndrome. What is the difference?

The answer is deceptively simple. If the car door rituals were Mark's only problem, he might well have OCD. But in combination with a variety of other difficulties, including avoiding eye contact, talking on and on about viruses, and showing no interest in friends, Asperger syndrome is a much more complete diagnosis. A label of OCD would account for Mark's problems only partially. People with OCD do not have trouble interacting and are able to converse with others in a very natural way. Other than their obsessions and compulsions, they display few unusual behaviors; it is *not*, for example, a feature of OCD to have special, highly focused interests (although this is widely misunderstood and probably accounts for many misdiagnoses). What distinguishes the autism spectrum disorders from all other conditions with which they might be confused are social reciprocity deficits and unusual communication style. If the hallmark symptoms of AS-HFA, as outlined in Table 1, are present, then the child has Asperger syndrome or high-functioning autism.

How do professionals decide if the child, in addition to AS-HFA, *also* has OCD? Most children and adolescents with OCD recognize that their behavior is unusual and experience it as intrusive and senseless. The majority of people with OCD are quite secretive about their rituals, realizing that other people would consider them bizarre. Indeed, the affected people themselves find the rituals bizarre and fervently wish they would go away. But try as they might to suppress them, they cannot stop themselves from performing the behavior. This is quite different from the experience of most children or adolescents with AS-HFA, who usually have little insight into the unusual nature of their behavior, do not consider it odd or eccentric, and make little attempt to conceal it. But not everyone with OCD has good insight into the unusual quality of their rituals; this is especially true of children. So a second important consideration in deciding whether a child has AS-HFA alone or both AS-HFA and OCD is the desire to achieve simplicity in diagnosis. Following the law of parsimony described above, most clinicians would not diagnose both conditions unless the manifestations of both were clearly present and the difficulties could not be accounted for by just one of the conditions.

A number of other disorders intersect with Asperger syndrome and high-functioning autism. In fact, OCD is not the most common misdiagnosis or partial diagnosis. Many children who are diagnosed with an autism spectrum disorder when they are somewhat older, after preschool, have received a previous diagnosis of attention-deficit/ hyperactivity disorder (ADHD). The hallmarks of this condition, as you may be aware and as the label conveys, are difficulty paying attention and controlling behavior and activity level. A child with ADHD may not seem to listen when spoken to or follow directions, may be reluctant to engage in tasks that are boring or effortful, may be distracted easily, fidget, leave his or her seat when sitting is expected, have difficulty waiting his or her turn, interrupt others, and talk excessively.

The similarities to autism spectrum disorders are probably immediately obvious. Many children with AS-HFA display every one of these problems, but often for very different reasons than the child with ADHD. The child with AS-HFA may not seem to listen and may not follow directions because of social deficits and language processing problems. He does not understand the centrality and importance of the human voice and does not orient to it naturally. Similarly, he may interrupt others, have trouble taking turns, and talk too much because of his difficulty reading social situations and knowing what is acceptable behavior in specific situations. He may be reluctant to do certain school assignments or have trouble staying seated, but not because these are inherently difficult tasks; they simply hold no interest for him. Praise from teachers or parents and high grades may not be incentives for the child with AS-HFA, who has a vastly different motivation and reinforcement system than that of the typical child. He may be distracted, but not usually by the noises and other goings-on that distract the child with ADHD: the child with AS-HFA is distracted by his own internal world, thoughts, and interests.

So one reason that children are often first diagnosed with ADHD, when in fact they have AS-HFA, is that there is some overlap between the symptoms of the two conditions. A second reason is that ADHD is a common disorder, and thus clinicians are often more aware of it and better trained in its diagnosis than in diagnosis of AS-HFA. Finally, the problems of ADHD (such as remaining seated, not waiting turns, and not following directions) may be more bothersome to teachers and parents, and thus may be more often brought to the attention of professionals than social awkwardness or highly specialized interests.

But just like a child with OCD alone, the child with ADHD alone does not have the problems with eye contact, conversation, range of interests, and imagination that the child with AS-HFA has. The same approach should be taken to distinguish AS-HFA from ADHD and the other conditions listed in Table 2 and to rule out any other apparently overlapping diagnosis. If the characteristic difficulties of AS-HFA are present, then the child has AS-HFA. The child receives multiple diagnoses only if all criteria for another condition are met and those features *cannot be accounted for by the AS-HFA diagnosis*. In Table 2, we have listed some conditions that are confused with AS-HFA.

The consequences of misdiagnosis can be serious. Obviously, it is important to know the true nature of your child's difficulties to understand her best, but accurate diagnosis is also critical to getting your child the best possible treatment. Certain treatments are designed specifically for AS-HFA and offer the best possible outcome in adult life (more on this in Chapter 4). An accurate diagnosis is essential to obtaining such resources. The correct diagnosis will also steer you away from interventions that will do no good and that might even harm your child, such as medications with serious side effects and behavioral treatments that focus on the wrong issues or make incorrect assumptions about the reasons that your child acts in the ways she does.

Table 2. Possible Previous Diagnoses, Incomplete Diagnoses, or Misdiagnoses

Diagnosis	Features
Attention-deficit/hyperactivity disorder	• Inattention • Hyperactivity • Impulsivity
Hearing impairment/deafness	• Reduced or complete lack of ability to hear sounds of multiple frequencies
Learning disabilities	• Difficulty in reading, spelling, mathematics, or written language that is unexpected given age, education, and intelligence
Mental retardation	• Intelligence scores below 70 • Inability to perform activities of daily living independently (for example, eat, dress, go to the toilet, communicate, work, play) and at levels expected for age
Nonverbal learning disability	• Math skills significantly below IQ • Nonverbal IQ significantly below Verbal IQ • Difficulty with spatial processes (puzzles, maps) • Poor handwriting • Poor motor skills; clumsiness
Obsessive–compulsive disorder	• Persistent, repetitive thoughts, actions or rituals • High anxiety if not allowed to perform acts • Understanding that the behavior is senseless
Oppositional defiant disorder	• Negativistic, hostile, defiant, or disobedient behavior toward authority figures
Reactive attachment disorder	• Markedly disturbed social relatedness • Significant abuse or neglect
Schizoid personality disorder	• Little interest in social relationships • Unemotional or few strong emotional responses
Schizophrenia or psychotic disorder	• Bizarre, fixed beliefs (delusions) • Unusual perceptual experiences (hallucinations) • Disorganized speech and behavior
Selective mutism	• Consistent failure to speak in social situations (for example, school) despite speaking in other situations (for example, home)

Diagnosis	Features
Social anxiety disorder (social phobia)	• Marked, persistent fear of social situations • Recognition that the fear is excessive/unreasonable
Speech–language disorders	• Failure to use pronunciation, vocabulary, or grammar (for example, tense, plurals) expected for age; shorter and less complex sentences. • Difficulty understanding language and processing verbal instructions
Tourette syndrome	• Tics (sudden, rapid, recurrent movements or sounds)

Is It Possible That My Child Has Something Else in Addition to AS-HFA?

Although we strive to achieve simplicity in diagnosis, it is not always possible or accurate to diagnose a child with AS-HFA alone. Having multiple psychiatric conditions is called "comorbidity," which is very important to detect, because if they are left untreated, these coexisting disorders can lead to an overall worsening in your child's functioning. Research has repeatedly shown that individuals with AS-HFA are at higher risk than other individuals for the conditions listed in Table 3, for reasons not fully understood yet. A study by Dr. Janet Lainhart, a child psychiatrist at the University of Utah, found that close to half of the adults with autism spectrum disorders she studied have one or more of these comorbid conditions. No studies on their prevalence in children have yet been conducted, but they are thought to be relatively common, especially by adolescence.

Professionals who are evaluating and treating children who may have AS-HFA have to tread a fine line between overdiagnosing many disorders and failing to spot true comorbidity. Children with AS-HFA often can't help in the diagnosis of a co-occurring condition because their self-awareness is limited and they have poor insight into their own emotions, difficulty reading their own and others' mental states, and limited ability to talk about abstract concepts. This is where parents and professionals who know the child well can step in. It may be up to you to spot and report any clear changes in behavior or thinking

Table 3. Other Disorders That Often Co-Occur with AS-HFA

Diagnosis	Features
Anxiety disorders	• Excessive worry • Avoidance of certain situations or objects due to fear
Attention-deficit/ hyperactivity disorder	• Inattention • Hyperactivity • Impulsivity
Depression	• Sadness and/or irritability • Loss of interest in previously pleasurable activities • Changes in eating and sleeping patterns • Fatigue and loss of energy • Feelings of worthlessness, hopelessness • Suicidal thoughts or behavior
Tourette syndrome	• Tics (sudden, rapid, recurrent movements or sounds)

in your child, which indicates the possibility of comorbidity. Autism does not cause bad moods, so if your previously happy child becomes irritable or tense or otherwise different in his moods for several weeks in a row, you may want to take him to a psychiatrist or a psychologist to explore whether depression or anxiety is complicating the AS-HFA. Similarly, if he or she suddenly develops a new behavior, such as injuring himself or being quite aggressive toward others, you should seriously consider a visit to your doctor. Finally, if your child does not respond to treatment interventions as you and your doctor expect, then you should examine whether there is more going on than AS-HFA alone. You should always raise the question of comorbidity at an initial assessment if you feel that your child's behavior doesn't fit the typical AS-HFA profile and you suspect there is more going on.

The Assessment Process

The exact sequence of events in the assessment process will vary depending on who does the evaluation and where. But let's start with the assumption that your child has been referred for an evaluation because you, a teacher, or someone else who has observed your child closely is concerned that a developmental problem may exist.

Who Is Qualified to Diagnose Autism Spectrum Conditions?

The types of professionals most often making such diagnoses are psychologists and psychiatrists, particularly those trained in childhood disorders. Other types of doctors, such as neurologists, pediatricians, and general practitioners (sometimes called "family practice doctors"), may also see your child for a diagnostic evaluation. Additionally, social workers are trained in the diagnostic process and how to use the DSM-IV, so they are qualified to make diagnoses. Other professionals, such as teachers, speech–language pathologists, and occupational therapists, may have some knowledge of autism and may well be the ones who first alert you to the possibility, but they are not trained in the diagnostic process. Since teachers and therapists often have experience with other children like your son or daughter, even though they cannot make a formal diagnosis, you would be wise to listen to their concerns and ask for a referral to a qualified professional. At some agencies, your child will be seen by a team of professionals from a wide variety of disciplines, including psychology, psychiatry, pediatrics, education, social work, and speech–language, so you and your child will get the benefit of even the professionals who are not, by themselves, able to make a diagnosis.

Whatever his or her particular credentials, the most important quality for your diagnostician is knowledge of and experience with autism spectrum disorders. It is not uncommon for professionals without such training, even those with appropriate degrees, to mistake the higher functioning autism spectrum disorders for something else. Just as you may have thought of a very remote, silent child obsessed with spinning objects in a corner when you heard the term "autism," so too many professionals without appropriate training think that a verbal, bright child who does not flap his hands cannot possibly have anything related to autism. This is likely what delayed both Lauren's and Clint's diagnoses. So be sure to ask, when scheduling an appointment for a diagnostic evaluation, if the examiner or team has expertise, or at least experience, with higher functioning autism spectrum disorders.

Developmental History

The two essential ingredients in a diagnostic evaluation are a thorough developmental history and an observation of your child. You, the par-

Are You Getting the Expert Help You Need for a Good Diagnosis?

Many different types of professionals are qualified to diagnose autism spectrum disorders. In our experience, expertise in the area of autism spectrum disorders is much more important to a thorough, accurate diagnosis than particular credentials. It can be difficult to know whether you have found the best person to evaluate your child, however, until you go through the process. Here are some questions to ask yourself as the evaluation proceeds. Any "no" answers should prompt you to ask the professional for an explanation, more information, or further evaluation. If you're not satisfied by the explanation, or you get a number of "no" answers, consider seeking another professional for a second opinion once the assessment is finished.

- Did the doctor interview you about your child's early history?

- Did the doctor spend at least 30 minutes with your child to observe his or her behavior?

- Did the doctor meet with you to explain the results of the assessment and answer your questions?

- Did the doctor's feedback seem to fit your child? Did the doctor understand the problems your child is experiencing that prompted you to seek the evaluation?

- Did the doctor explain which diagnosis best fits your child and why?

- Did the doctor give you options for treatment that are available in your community and specific referrals (phone numbers, and the like)?

- Did the doctor provide or promise to provide a report that summarizes the results of your child's testing?

ents, tell the professionals in detail what your child is like at home, on a day-to-day basis, since some of both her strengths and her difficulties might not be apparent during the observation period. Autism spectrum disorders involve two different kinds of symptoms: (1) typical behaviors that fail to develop (for example, empathy, close friendships, pretend play, and eye contact) and (2) unusual behaviors that are not present in other children (for example, echoing from videos, obsessive interests, or extreme anxiety over changes in routine). The evaluator will ask you specific questions about these behaviors, both what they are like at the present time and how they were when your child was young, before age 5.

Observation of Your Child

The professional will also observe your child and interact with her for some period of time, making note of the same types of symptoms he or she asked you about in the interview. The examiner might set up specific situations to make sure that certain symptoms, if present, are evident during the observation period. Eye contact, for example, is often poor in children with autism spectrum conditions. To be certain that your child's eye contact is limited with the examiner because of an autism spectrum disorder and not just due to shyness or lack of opportunity, the examiner might set up explicit scenarios that powerfully pull for eye contact, such as making it necessary that your child ask for help. In such situations, typical children almost always make eye contact. Similarly, the examiner might ask your child to tell a familiar story, because most typical children will periodically make eye contact to be sure that you are following them or are interested in what they are saying. An experienced evaluator might engineer a specific opportunity for your child to empathize with him or her to examine this criterion accurately. He might pretend to stub his toe or shut his finger in the door or might mention that something sad happened to him recently (such as that his favorite pet was lost) to gauge your child's reaction and ability to offer comfort or support to others.

In most cases, the parent interview and direct observation of your child are enough for the examiner to make or rule out the autism spectrum diagnoses. As may already be apparent, there is no *medical* test for autism spectrum conditions. We cannot draw blood and look at chromosomes or levels of any particular chemicals to tell us if your child has Asperger syndrome or high-functioning autism. We can take pictures of his brain (for example, with magnetic resonance imaging [MRI] scans), but that won't tell us his diagnosis. As you will read in Chapter 3, we have found a few brain abnormalities in some people with autism and Asperger syndrome but nothing present in all (even most) AS-HFA people or not present in some non-AS-HFA people. So currently there are no specific biological tests for the autism spectrum disorders. Professionals rely on the presence of the specific behaviors described in this chapter to diagnose the conditions. But this is not necessarily the problem it may sound like. All disorders in the DSM-IV are diagnosed on the basis of behavior (rather than biology), and the autism spectrum disorders happen to have among the very highest reliability of these disorders. That means that if several different professionals were to see the same child with AS-HFA, they would be more likely to agree on his diagnosis than were they to see a child with another (less reliable) diagnosis, such as ADHD.

Medical Tests: Informative but Not Usually Diagnostic

A related question you may have is whether specific medical tests might be helpful in your child's evaluation, even though they might not be critical to making the actual diagnosis. The answer to this question varies from child to child. Some children have certain risk factors or events in their history that make a full medical work-up highly desirable. For example, approximately 25% of children with autism spectrum disorders also have seizures, which can range from short blackouts to violent convulsions of the entire body. Seizures are most common in more classically autistic children, but can also occur in individuals with AS-HFA. The most common periods in which seizures start are preschool and adolescence. If your child has ever displayed behaviors indicative of potential seizures, then neurological testing, such as an electroencephalogram (EEG) and/or an MRI (brain scan), may be ordered by your doctor. If your child went through a stage of development in which he or she lost skills (for example, learning to talk and then losing the ability to speak), neurological testing may again be warranted. All children should have genetic testing, because in a minority of cases AS-HFA is associated with identifiable genetic conditions such as Fragile X syndrome. If your child has anything slightly unusual about his face, hands, feet, or skin, he should be seen by a medical doctor. For example, if he has multiple brown or white birthmarks on his skin, large or unusually shaped ears, or other minor differences in how he looks, he may have a genetic condition that underlies his autism that might require additional medical treatment and genetic counseling. If other members of your family, including your siblings, nieces, nephews, and other children, have been slow or unusual in their development, this may warrant seeing a geneticist for genetic counseling.

Psychological Tests

Just as there are medical tests that are not diagnostic, but that are informative, so also there are behavioral or psychological tests that are not needed for the diagnosis but nevertheless can be very helpful in painting a complete picture of your child's strengths, weaknesses, treatment needs, and so forth. Probably the most common additional psychological testing that will be done during a diagnostic evaluation is an intelligence (or IQ) test.

Intelligence Tests

For verbal children over age 5, the test that is used most often is the Wechsler Intelligence Scale for Children, or WISC (pronounced "whisk"). It provides three different IQ scores, one measuring verbal intelligence, another measuring nonverbal intelligence, and a third combined score. The WISC, like the DSM, is revised periodically, both to improve its reliability and to update its norms. It is currently in its third edition and so is known as the WISC-III ("whisk-three"). If your child is over age 17, he or she may have been given the adult version, the Wechsler Adult Intelligence Scale, Third Edition (or WAIS-III, pronounced "wace-three"). If your child is under age 6, a variety of different tests may be used, including the Wechsler Preschool and Primary Scale of Intelligence (WPPSI-III, pronounced "wipsy-three"), the Mullen Scales of Early Learning, the Stanford–Binet Intelligence Scale, the Leiter International Performance Scale, and others. If your child has taken one of these tests within a year or so, perhaps at school, the evaluator may just review the scores, rather than retesting the child now (this has an added financial advantage, as testing done through the school is free). Be sure to bring any records of earlier testing to your appointment so that your doctor can use these previous scores whenever possible.

It's often useful to know the broad range in which your child's intelligence falls so you can plan the most appropriate educational interventions. It is probably a good idea, however, to view your child's IQ scores with some caution. Children with autism spectrum disorders often have attention and motivation problems that prevent them from scoring well on IQ tests. Furthermore, IQ scores reflect the "average" of all the different subtests that are given, and children with autism spectrum disorders often show greatly varying levels of ability across the subtests. Thus, the average score may not be that meaningful as a true reflection of your child's abilities. IQ test scores need to be interpreted in light of the child's behavior during the test itself. They may also change as your child gets older and becomes better (or worse) at taking IQ tests. And you need to know what the three different scores indicate. The individual verbal and nonverbal IQ scores should not be viewed as absolute indications of your child's intellectual potential. Even the overall combined score should be considered within the broader context of your child's behavior and accomplishments in everyday living, which are also measures of intelligence. But in the case of children with AS-HFA, IQ scores may be even less accurate than in typical children who don't have some difficulty communicating and relating to others. Due to social difficulties, for example, your child might not care about the examiner's reinforcement ("You're working hard") and thus not be motivated to perform her best on the IQ test. Or his unusual style of speaking might be an obstacle on certain tests. For example, when asked to define the word "glove," a child with Asperger syndrome might say, "a hand covering not in fashion these days unless it is a cold season" rather than give the more typical answer, "something you wear on your hands when it is cold." The first definition is not among the options for correct answers in the IQ test manual and therefore would not receive full credit. For these reasons we advise all parents, but parents of children with AS-HFA in particular, to pay more attention to the *range* of functioning that your child's score falls into, rather than the specific number. You may be told, for example, that your child is functioning in the "average" range, the "superior" range, or the "borderline" range. The average score on all IQ tests is 100. Children obtaining scores below 70 are considered mentally retarded. Those with scores from 70 to 80 fall in the borderline range, from 80 to 90 in the low average range, from 90 to 110 in the average range, from 110 to 120 in the high average range, from 120 to 130 in the superior range, and above 130 in the very superior range. So if your child is on the low end of the average range, he or she may well need extra help in school (more on this in Chapter 7). Certain IQ patterns also may indicate learning disabilities and the need for further testing.

As mentioned earlier, you will probably be given at least three IQ scores by the examiner interpreting the results. All are on the same scale just described (with an average of 100). The Verbal IQ score indicates how well your child performed on tests that require language— for example, defining words, remembering lists of numbers, and describing how two things are related. The Performance IQ score measures how well your child carries out tasks that don't require language but rely on visual–spatial skills, such as putting together puzzles, finding the way out of mazes, and putting cards in order to tell a coherent story. These two scores can be combined into a Full Scale IQ score that indicates your child's *overall* functioning across both verbal and nonverbal tasks. Sometimes your child's three scores will be similar, indicating that he or she is equally good at verbal and nonverbal tasks, but other times they can be quite different, with your child performing very highly on one kind of test, but much more poorly on another kind. In such situations, the overall Full Scale score will fall somewhere in between the two extremes. Some research suggests that children with Asperger syndrome tend to have higher Verbal than Performance IQs, while children with high-functioning autism show the opposite pattern. This is, however, by no means a universal pattern. Some children with Asperger syndrome have very good visual–spatial skills that are better developed than their language, some children with high-functioning autism have high Verbal IQ and lower Performance IQ, and some children with each condition show no differences between Verbal and Performance skills. This is why you won't find particular IQ patterns included in the diagnostic criteria. It's also why you should not be concerned if your child has one diagnosis but demonstrates the other IQ pattern. This does not mean the diagnosis is wrong.

Additional Tests

Your child's evaluation may also include educational testing that examines how well he or she reads, spells, performs math calculations, writes, and so on; speech–language testing; neuropsychological testing that looks at memory, fine motor skills, spatial processing, and the like; a nutritional evaluation; and many other things, depending on how comprehensive the team conducting the evaluation is. All these areas are of some interest in that they produce the most complete picture of your child, but parents and professionals sometimes have to weigh the desire to be comprehensive with practical constraints, such as finances. If the professional is appropriately trained, a relatively quick evaluation that includes only a parent interview and an observation of your child and contains none of these "extras" can still provide an accurate diagnosis. The signs of autism spectrum disorders are readily discernable to the experienced professional who has asked the right questions and noticed the right aspects of behavior, without any additional intellectual, neurological, or educational testing. Be sure to ask the doctor or team assessing your child how many children with autism they see. Or call your state autism society to obtain a referral to an experienced professional. The Internet also contains websites that include lists of qualified doctors by state.

After the Diagnosis

When they first receive a diagnosis of high-functioning autism or Asperger syndrome, parents experience a wide range of reactions, from one extreme of shock, grief, or denial to another extreme of relief and even happiness. More commonly, there is a mixture of negative and positive feelings. Many parents have known for a long time that there was something different about their child and have actively sought an explanation, but still hope that nothing is really wrong and their fears will prove unfounded. Parents worry about the stigma of a label, about the future, and about their child's ability to live independently and be happy. They wonder if they need to change their expectations for their child or treat him or her differently. But with a diagnosis comes the promise of intervention and support. If a condition is common enough to have a name, then perhaps there is something known about how to treat it. And there must be others with this condition! You will meet other parents who know exactly what you are going through and who have great ideas about how to live with and enjoy AS-HFA in your family. You will come to understand why your child does what he or she does, what motivates him or her, what tickles him or her, what is hard for him or her, and why. With a diagnosis comes some ability to share his or her perspective and see the world through the eyes of your special child. Two mothers now share their stories:

"It's a week after Charlie's third birthday, and I've gathered our extended family on our back porch to hear directly from a neurologist the diagnosis and prognosis for him. I'm exhausted from running around to different specialists and libraries looking for answers or clues to Charlie's behavior and explaining to our family that his issues are not just speech-related, nor will he just outgrow them. I'm tired of being the one with answers and being challenged on my assumptions by caring family members who only see Charlie occasionally or who have more anecdotes on child development than facts. I want them to hear it directly from a nationally recognized doctor. Maybe now, with the same base of information, we can all start working together to get Charlie the help he needs and stop arguing about what it is. The doctor is ready to start. He says, 'Charlie has Asperger syndrome' and goes on with information about the disorder and what we can expect in the future. But I've stopped listening. Although I've searched for this answer for a year, my heart is so totally overwhelmed with grief at the pain I fear Charlie will face all his life and the greater fear that I won't be able to do enough to help him that I hear no more."

"Timmy turned 7 the day we received the diagnosis of high-functioning autism. Finally, the exhaustive search to discover what made our son so different—so special—had ended. A sense of relief overwhelmed us. At last, we had the answer, the answer that would give purpose and direction to our long journey. Now we could focus all our efforts on learning everything possible about autism. Now our doctors and therapists would have a unified goal. We had traveled far, but our journey had really only just begun. We felt almost joyful. The doctor thought we were crazy."

What Should I Tell My Child?

Parents often ask about sharing the news with their child. The first issue is usually "*Should* we tell him [or her]?" The answer to this question depends very much on the child's age, temperament, and other life circumstances, but usually the answer is "Yes, at some point." The next question, then, is *when*? The best way to determine if your child is ready to hear about AS-HFA is if he or she is expressing awareness of his or her differences, particularly voicing concerns, as when Joseph says "I'm a geek" to his parents. Almost all the children we diagnose are highly aware that they are different from others. Some are concerned, like Joseph, while others are not, but most can readily articulate that they are unlike other kids. Many children with AS-HFA attribute this to some terrible flaw. "I have a bad brain," one boy told the first author (S.O.). After harboring hidden fears about himself for so long, finding out about AS-HFA was a tremendous relief for this child. He heard that, yes, he is different, but his differences are very special. They include things he is really good at, as well as a few things he is not so good at but for which help is available.

This brings us to the third issue: *how* to share the news. The following is relevant for telling not only your child, but also siblings, grandparents, friends, and neighbors, about AS-HFA (more about disclosing diagnosis in adulthood appears in Chapter 9). It is critical that the way the diagnosis is framed be positive, emphasizing your child's strengths and special skills. In discussing the difficulties that are part of AS-HFA, we often find it helpful to compare it to a learning disability. You can ask your child if he or she knows anyone who has trouble with reading, or math, or paying attention and staying seated. Emphasize that most of us have weaknesses of some sort or another; some people wear glasses, others walk with a cane, others are slow readers, others are very clumsy on the playground. But those people aren't bad at everything; there are many things they can do well. You might say, "The girl in your class who can't read well can do math just fine, has lots of friends, and is good at sports. You, with AS-HFA, are like that too. You have trouble making friends, looking others in the eye, and knowing what to say in a conversation [choose the specific difficulties your child has that he is aware of]. But you have a great memory, you are the best speller in your class, you are good with computers, and you know so much about certain fascinating topics." Help your child understand that diversity is wonderful and that it is highly desirable to have people who are "different" among us. (There is a very helpful appendix in Liane Willey's book, *Pretending to Be Normal*, on explaining AS-HFA to other people; choosing who, when, and how to share this news; and dealing with reactions.)

Begin the process of embracing the characteristics of AS-HFA, for both your child and you. For this is who your child is. Take away the symptoms of AS-HFA, and your special, unique, and much-loved child would be gone. You will learn that living with AS-HFA can have many challenges, but also great rewards that are uniquely yours to cherish.

CHAPTER 3

Causes of Autism Spectrum Disorders

Seth had experienced many, many ear infections and chest colds as an infant and young child. He seemed to be constantly sick and was in the pediatrician's office almost weekly. His mother has always wondered if this had anything to do with his autism.

Chad had seemed like a perfectly normal baby until a few months before his second birthday, when he stopped saying the few words he had been learning and seemed to lose interest in other people. Later, his family wondered if his 18-month vaccinations had had anything to do with his PDDNOS. He developed a high fever after the shots and cried inconsolably for 2 days. Were the two related?

Lauren's mother had had an extremely difficult pregnancy. She had high blood pressure and was placed on total bed rest for 6 weeks. Her amniotic fluid levels were low and the baby rarely moved. Her doctor was worried about fetal distress, and induced labor with Pitocin a month early. Lauren was born weighing only 5 pounds. She required resuscitation at birth and remained hospitalized, on oxygen, for 2 weeks. Could these complications really be just a coincidence or were they related to Lauren's difficulties?

Scientists do not yet have complete answers to these questions, but very strong evidence suggests that the autism spectrum disorders are biological in origin and not caused by parenting or other psycho-social environmental causes. Differences in the size and organization of the brain, as well as in how it works, in individuals with autism spectrum disorders versus normal individuals have been found. Autism spectrum disorders and related difficulties also run in families, so we think that genetic factors also play a role. This chapter summarizes what we know so far about the causes of autism spectrum disorders. It's important to understand that most of the studies conducted to date were done on individuals with autism. The few studies conducted on the causes of Asperger syndrome suggest that the roots of the two conditions are similar; thus, even though more research is needed, much of what we summarize here about autism is applicable to Asperger syndrome too.

Brain Differences in Autism Spectrum Disorders

When Dr. Kanner first described autism in 1943, he wrote that children with the disorder were born with an "innate," or inborn, difficulty bonding with people. In the mid-20th century, most doctors were trained in the psychoanalytic tradition, which attributed all behavioral and mental disorders to early childhood experiences. Thus autism was suspected to be caused by the social environment rather than by biology. Dr. Kanner was influenced by these ideas. Later he and others blamed autism on parents. They described "refrigerator mothers" who were so emotionally cold and rejecting that they caused their children to retreat into an autistic "cocoon" of safety. This view began to lose credibility in the 1960s, however, after Dr. Bernard Rimland published *Infantile Autism: The Syndrome and Its Implications for a Neural Theory of Behavior*. In this 1964 book the author attacked parent causation theories and pointed out that there was absolutely no research data to support them. He was the first to suggest that autism was due to differences in how the brain worked. This suggestion has stimulated a good deal of research into possible brain differences in individuals with autism spectrum disorders.

To understand where the information collected to date comes from, you need a rudimentary grasp of the methods used to study the brain. *Structural imaging* takes pictures of brain anatomy or structures to see if anything is grossly abnormal (that is, much smaller or bigger than average, in the wrong place, or missing altogether). Specific structural imaging techniques include computed tomography (CT) scans and magnetic resonance imaging (MRI) scans. These techniques differ in how they take pictures of the brain and how much detail they can provide. CT is an older technology that is less often used today. *Postmortem or autopsy studies* examine the brains of people who have died. This method permits scientists to look at the brain in a much more detailed manner than CT or MRI. Researchers are actually able to examine individual brain cells (called neurons) rather than the large structures, composed of millions of neurons, captured by CT and MRI. Autopsy work takes a long time and is very difficult for a number of reasons, but it provides important information that is not available through any other means. *Functional imaging*, the newest technology available to examine the brain, looks specifically at how the brain *works*. Scientists can study whether when certain behaviors are performed or tasks completed, the same parts of the brain are active (and working as hard and as efficiently) in individuals with autism spectrum disorders as they are in persons without these disorders. Figure 1 illustrates the major structures of the brain and how they affect social behavior.

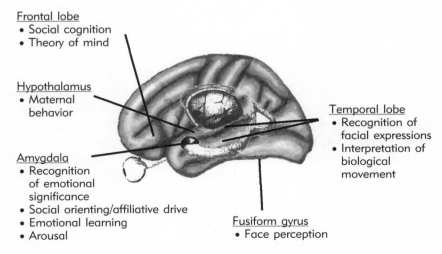

Frontal lobe
- Social cognition
- Theory of mind

Hypothalamus
- Maternal behavior

Amygdala
- Recognition of emotional significance
- Social orienting/affiliative drive
- Emotional learning
- Arousal

Temporal lobe
- Recognition of facial expressions
- Interpretation of biological movement

Fusiform gyrus
- Face perception

Figure 1. Social brain systems. Adapted from Schultz and Klin (in press) by permission of Robert T. Schultz.

Autopsy Studies

Only a few investigations of this type have been done, since they are so difficult to perform and since it is uncommon both for individuals with autism spectrum disorders to die prematurely (thankfully) and for their survivors to donate their brains to science. The few studies that have been done have found two types of brain abnormalities. First, they have found that there are too many brain cells (neurons) in a region known as the *limbic system*, which lies deep in the center of the brain and is important to social and emotional behavior. Moreover, the cells are smaller and more tightly packed together than they are supposed to be. This may mean that they do not have the correct shape and/or enough room to make the connections with other brain cells that allow them to function as they should. Autopsy investigations have also revealed significantly fewer brain cells in another part of the brain called the *cerebellum*, which is important in both motor coordination and cognitive activities. While these findings are very interesting, they were based on the study of relatively few brains (approximately 25) and were not found in all the brains examined. Thus we are not sure how widespread these brain differences are in people with autism spectrum disorders. Additionally, almost all the brains studied came from individuals with severe autism and mental retardation, and in some cases epilepsy, and thus we are not yet sure if these results pertain to children or adolescents with higher functioning autism spectrum disorders.

Structural Imaging Studies

This research method has found a wide variety of abnormalities. In all brains (autistic and nonautistic) there are spaces, known as *ventricles*, that contain fluid instead of brain tissue. Some studies have found that the ventricles are larger than normal in some people with autism, which may mean that brain tissue around the ventricles has been lost. This finding is not specific to autism, however; it has been found in a variety of other syndromes. It appears to be a marker for an abnormal brain, rather than specific to autism.

Dr. Eric Courchesne, a prominent neuroscientist at the University of California at San Diego, reported in the late 1980s that a very specific part of the cerebellum (called the *vermis*, which is the Latin word for worm, because of its shape) was smaller in many people with autism.

Some more recent studies have confirmed this finding, while others have not. Recent investigations have shown that this part of the cerebellum is abnormal in people without autism too. Children with leukemia who have undergone radiation treatment often have a vermis smaller than normal, as do some children with psychosis (a condition involving bizarre behavior that appears out of touch with reality) and children with certain genetic syndromes.

Both imaging and autopsy studies have demonstrated that about one-quarter of individuals with autism spectrum disorders have larger than average brains (and heads). Just as with the limbic and cerebellar findings reported above, however, this finding does not appear specific to autism. Moreover, how it might cause autistic behavior is not understood. During normal brain growth and development, there is at first a period of tremendous overproduction of neurons: the brain grows more cells than it really needs. Later, those neurons that aren't being used much or that haven't made important connections to other areas of the brain are weeded out. Some scientists believe that the large size of brains in some individuals with autism spectrum disorders indicates that this "pruning" mechanism has failed. This might mean that there is more background "noise" (or static) in the brain, which prevents it from functioning most efficiently. This is currently only a hypothesis, and we do not yet know what causes the brain to be larger or how this directly affects the way the brain functions.

Functional Imaging and Other Studies of How the Brain Works

Two specific areas of the brain have been the focus of investigations into whether the brains of those with autism spectrum disorders work differently from the brains of those without autism spectrum disorders.

Frontal Lobes

Since autism spectrum disorders always involve social deficits and repetitive behaviors, the areas of the brain that control these functions have been a focus of neuroimaging studies. In the late 1970s, two American neurologists, Drs. Antonio Damasio and Ralph Maurer, published a paper that pointed out behavioral similarities between people with autism and patients with damage to their *frontal lobes* (the region in the front of the brain, just behind our eyes and forehead). Both groups had difficulty controlling their emotions, would get very upset by small changes, were compulsive (wanting things "just so"), and were rigid in their solutions to problems, seeing things in a concrete, black-and-white manner. This led to a theory, still influential today, that if the frontal lobes did not develop correctly, this could cause autism. So far, however, no evidence of abnormalities in the size, shape, or placement of frontal structures has been found. Functional imaging studies have, however, found a variety of problems in how the frontal lobes work. For example, for individuals with autism spectrum disorders, there is both less blood flow to and less electrical activity in this region, suggesting that their frontal lobes are not as active as they are supposed to be. In normal people, it is typical that multiple brain regions are needed to perform a task. Some studies of individuals with autism spectrum disorders have found that the activity of the frontal lobes is not well coordinated with other parts of the brain during task performance. Studies of normal volunteers and people with frontal damage have shown us that the frontal lobes are important to planning, flexibility, organization, behavioral control, and reasoning. If they are not working as efficiently or as well as they should, this could explain some symptoms of autism spectrum disorders.

Medial Temporal Lobes

The second region of specific interest in autism is the *temporal lobes*, which lie on the sides of the brain, roughly at the level of the ears. The specific part of the temporal lobes that seems to be involved is their very inner lining, lying closest to the center of the brain. This region is known as the *medial* (or middle) *temporal lobes* and includes the limbic system, which we discussed earlier with regard to autopsy studies. Some of the structures in this area include the amygdala and the hippocampus. This region is important to emotional expression and regulation, the understanding and decoding of information that we see in other people's faces, social behavior, and memory. Experiments in animals have shown that when this region is damaged, severe social impairments, isolation, and stereotyped, self-stimulatory behaviors result. Some, but not all, autopsy and structural MRI studies have shown differences in the amygdala (for example, being smaller than normal or having too many small, densely packed neurons) and other medial temporal structures in some people with autism spectrum disorders. Studies conducted by one of us (G.D.), as well as others, have shown that individuals with autism do in fact have problems in processing basic aspects of social information, including face recognition and discrimination of facial expressions—processing that is controlled by parts of the limbic system and temporal lobes.

In a study published in 2000, Dr. Simon Baron-Cohen and his colleagues measured brain function (using an imaging technique known as functional MRI, or fMRI) while people with and without autism spectrum disorders looked at pictures of eyes. Their job was to decide what emotion the eyes conveyed. These researchers found that adults without autism spectrum disorders relied heavily on both the amygdala and the frontal lobes to perform this task. In other words, these two regions seemed to be most important to processing the social and emotional information conveyed by the eyes. In contrast, adults with either high-functioning autism or Asperger syndrome used the frontal lobes much less than the normal adults and did not "turn on" the amygdala at all when looking at the pictures of eyes. Instead, they used other parts of the brain that are normally not active during this task. Another study, led by Dr. Robert Schultz at Yale University, found that people with autism and Asperger syndrome used the part of the brain that normally makes sense of objects when they looked at faces. Dawson and colleagues recently discovered that some very young (3- to 4-year-old) children with autism fail to show recognition of a mother's face, but show normal recognition of familiar objects. The brain systems responsible for face recognition come on line very early in life, offering the possibility that face recognition impairment may turn out to be one of the earliest indicators of abnormal brain development in autism. These findings don't mean that your child does not recognize you. Instead, they suggest that your child may rely on cues other than facial features for recognition (such as touch and voice).

These findings suggest that one reason people with autism may make less eye contact and may have so much more trouble understanding others' emotions, thoughts, and intentions is that critical regions of the brain are not working when they should be. Even when people with autism spectrum disorders can figure out what someone's eyes or face conveys, they do so in a different way than everyone else, which may be less efficient or take more time. The medial temporal area of the brain is being investigated by research teams around the world and may turn out to be one (but probably not the only) region that is abnormal in autism spectrum disorders. Indeed, as you can see in the picture of the brain on page 58, many areas of the brain are involved in social behavior. Researchers are actively discovering which parts of this complex system do not functioning properly and therefore account for the difficulty that those with autism spectrum disorders have in relating socially.

Brain Changes in Asperger Syndrome

Very few studies have specifically examined brain differences in individuals with Asperger syndrome and how (or if) they differ from those of individuals with autism. In the amygdala study done by Baron-Cohen, no differences were found between adults with high-functioning autism and those with Asperger syndrome, suggesting that the amygdala may be a structure involved in all autism spectrum conditions. Other recent research has found abnormalities in the brains of individuals with Asperger syndrome that are similar to those reported in individuals with autism, including enlargement of the ventricles, decreased frontal activity, missing tissue in the frontal lobes, and smaller than normal medial temporal, limbic, and cerebellar structures. Most of these studies have been case reports of only one or two people with Asperger syndrome, so the numbers are very small and we cannot be certain how representative they are of most people with Asperger syndrome.

As mentioned in Chapter 2, some research has found that individuals with Asperger syndrome have trouble with visual–spatial tasks, like puzzles and maps. This led to the hypothesis that the right side (or hemisphere) of the brain, which controls such abilities, is dysfunctional in individuals with Asperger syndrome, while the left side of the brain, which controls language functions, is affected in people with classic autism. This is an appealing theory, for if research proved it to be true, it would clearly show that Asperger syndrome and autism are distinct conditions because they result from different types of brain dysfunction. Unfortunately, however, this theory is probably too good to be true. It has long been evident that classically autistic children have difficulty with right hemisphere functions too, such as voice intonation and rhythm and the understanding of facial expressions and emotions. Recent studies have found both right and left hemisphere abnormalities in individuals with Asperger syndrome. And researchers from Yale University found no differences in the MRI scans of people with high-functioning autism, people with Asperger syndrome, and people with PDDNOS. This study looked only at the cerebellum and other structures in the back of the brain and did not examine the amygdala, medial temporal or frontal lobes, or the right or left hemispheres. Therefore, while the studies summarized in this section suggest, as a whole, that the brain abnormalities in individuals with Asperger syndrome and individuals with high-functioning autism may be similar, it is too early to form conclusions. More research is desperately needed.

Summary

The field has come a long way since parents were considered to be the cause of autism spectrum disorders. Study after study finds brain differences in people with autism and Asperger syndrome, although no signature autistic anomaly, one that is close to universal and specific to the autism spectrum disorders, has yet been found. This may, at first glance, be disappointing and perhaps even surprising, given the clear impairment that autism spectrum disorders can cause. Yet autism spectrum disorders have many faces, with some people being high functioning and others being mentally retarded, some being highly verbal while others do not use language at all, some having severe problem behaviors (for example, aggression, screaming, destructiveness) while others have no sign of such difficulties. Failing to control for all these differences among people with autism spectrum disorders and to study fairly pure samples may well explain the contradictory results of previous studies. In addition, many of the investigations reviewed above did not take into account the mental handicap of many people with autism, possibly meaning these results are applicable only to people with autism spectrum disorders who are significantly impaired.

Many scientists suspect that the brain differences found so far are not necessarily the ones that are central to generating autistic symptoms. The sophistication of imaging tools is increasing rapidly, but has likely not yet reached anything close to their eventual capacity. The techniques used a decade ago, when much of the research just reported was performed, were far less powerful and may have been able to identify only the most obvious brain differences. The next decade holds great promise for finding more answers about the brain differences in people with autism spectrum disorders and how they cause the conditions. In contrast, much progress has already been made in understanding how genes may contribute to the development of autism spectrum disorders.

Genetic Influences in the Autism Spectrum Disorders

Even after the terribly wrong theories that parents caused autism had been put to rest, most scientists dismissed the idea that genetic factors might play any role in the development of autism. For one thing, it was extremely rare that a child with autism had a parent with autism, a pattern that we usually expect to see in a genetic condition. Occasionally, an autistic child would have a brother or sister who also had autism, but this again was considered too uncommon to support a genetic explanation. In the 1970s, two eminent psychiatrists questioned this logic. Sir Michael Rutter is a famous British child psychiatrist who was knighted by the queen of England for his important research contributions to the understanding of autism and other childhood disorders. Dr. Susan Folstein is a prominent child psychiatrist in the United States who has published many papers on the genetics of autism. Both scientists reasoned that since the social difficulties of autism remain in adulthood, someone with autism is unlikely to marry and have children. Obviously, then, there would be few families with both an affected child and an affected parent. And while the rate of autism in siblings was small, it was much, much higher than the rate in the general population. These realizations led to the birth of a new field, the study of genetic contributions to autism. There is now very strong evidence that in many (but perhaps not all) families, genetics plays some role in the development of the condition. Unfortunately, it is already abundantly clear that untangling the genetics of autism will not be simple. Multiple genes appear to be involved in causing the disorder, and some families seem to carry different genes from other families. It also appears that the genes have broader effects than just autism itself. A variety of different problems seem to run in the families of children with autism spectrum conditions that may all be caused by the same genes. Thus, autism is just one of several possible outcomes of having these genes. For these reasons, genetic counseling for the autism spectrum disorders, even if and when we know all the genes involved in causing the conditions, will be complex. We are very far away from being able to provide families with information about the risk involved in future pregnancies. Again, however, we have made significant strides.

The first tip that autism might have some genetic basis came when Drs. Rutter and Folstein realized that the risk of having a second child with the condition, while still low (about 3–5%), was actually much higher than the risk if you'd never had a child with autism (about 6 chances in 1,000, or 0.6%). Noticing that a condition "runs in families" does not conclusively prove that it is genetic, however. A second piece of evidence came from twin studies, which found that the likelihood that twins would both have autism was much higher if the twins were *identical*, that is, shared all their genes, than if they were *fraternal*, that is, shared on average only about half of their genes. Research showed that if a fraternal twin had autism, the chance that the co-twin would also be diagnosed with it was less than 10%. In contrast, if an identical twin was diagnosed with autism, then the chance that the co-twin would also be affected was over 60%. Studies also showed that while many co-twins had full-blown autism, others demonstrated language, cognitive, or social difficulties that fell short of an autism spectrum diagnosis but were nevertheless quite impairing. Many scientists now believe that the genes involved do not cause autism itself but instead cause a variety of language and social differences and personality styles, of which autism is the extreme form.

Some children with known genetic disorders have autism, providing another piece of evidence that autism can have genetic origins. Fragile X syndrome and tuberous sclerosis are two genetic conditions that are readily diagnosed through genetic testing. The specific mutations in DNA that cause the conditions are known, and it is possible to diagnose both disorders before a child is born and to counsel couples who carry the genetic mutations for future pregnancies. A proportion of children with both fragile X syndrome and tuberous sclerosis develop autistic symptoms,[1] suggesting that the genes involved in causing these disorders may also be involved in causing autism.

....

[1]However, only a very small proportion of children with autism spectrum disorders have either fragile X syndrome or tuberous sclerosis. Some doctors routinely screen all autistic children for these conditions, but others suggest genetic testing only if the child with autism has certain physical features common in fragile X syndrome or tuberous sclerosis, as mentioned in Chapter 2.

In the 1990s, the Human Genome Project, an international collaboration to map all human genes to specific locations on chromosomes, made it possible to home in on parts of the genome most likely to contain genes for autism. *Linkage analysis* is a type of genetic research in which scientists study how closely "linked" certain diseases or traits are with certain regions of specific chromosomes. Linkage analysis does not tell us exactly which gene or genes within the region are responsible for the disease, but it does tell us which parts of which chromosomes may contain important genes. Recently, a region on the long arm[2] of chromosome 7 has demonstrated linkage with autism in a very large European study. In addition, a region on the long arm of chromosome 15, in which genetic material is duplicated and the second copy of the DNA is inserted backward (known as an inverted duplication), has been identified in between 1% and 4% of autistic participants in several research studies. Thus, some of the genes leading to autism may be on chromosomes 7 and 15. So far, however, this knowledge has few practical benefits. We do not yet know which specific genes are involved, nor do we know what the genes do or how they cause autism. Presumably, the genes are important for brain development, particularly development of those brain regions that contribute to normal social and communication ability, but the route from genes to behavior is still far from clear.

There appear to be a variety of traits that run in the families of people with autism and Asperger syndrome, especially related to the areas of language and social abilities. Higher rates of language delay, articulation problems, learning difficulties, social difficulties, and social anxiety are more often found in relatives of people with autism than in family members of people with other disabilities, such as Down syndrome. Studies indicate that these milder difficulties show up in about 10–20% of siblings of individuals with autism and often in parents as well.

The strengths of people with autism and Asperger syndrome can run in their families too. Parents and siblings often have similar talents and interests as those of people with autism spectrum disorders. British researcher Simon Baron-Cohen proposed a theory that people in families with a member with an autism spectrum disorder would be es-

---

[2]Chromosomes are shaped like an X, but the intersection is not in the middle of the X; it is displaced toward the top of the X, thus yielding two "long arms" on the bottom and two "short arms" on the top.

pecially skilled at understanding mechanical objects (such as how machines work), physical cause-and-effect mechanisms, and visual–spatial problems (as in puzzles). He and others have tested the theory that not only characteristic difficulties but also characteristic strengths run in families. Dr. Baron-Cohen's team found that the parents of children with autism or Asperger syndrome were more likely to be engineers, physicists, and mathematicians than the parents of other children (other scientists have also found elevated rates of accounting and science careers in families of individuals with autism spectrum disorders). Dr. Baron-Cohen's research group also surveyed over a thousand university students majoring either in literature or in math, physics, or engineering. They found that the rate of autism spectrum disorders was significantly higher in the families of the math, physics, or engineering students than in the families of the literature students. Finally, this British group of researchers tested the parents of children with autism spectrum disorders directly, giving them tests of both social understanding and visual-spatial skill. They found that the parents of students with autism spectrum disorders were more skilled at solving puzzles and finding hidden shapes in complex drawings than control parents, as well as slightly less accurate than the other parents at interpreting the expressions on people's faces. Some more recent research projects have confirmed the finding that strong visual–spatial, mechanical, and memory skills are often found in the families of individuals with autism spectrum disorders.

These findings all converge on one conclusion. What appears to be genetically transmitted in the families of people with autism spectrum disorders is not an autism spectrum disorder per se, but a certain distinctive style of thinking, relating, and reacting to the world that brings with it both limitations and strengths. This underscores the future limits we envision in the ability to provide genetic counseling. If a person carries certain genes, it does not necessarily mean that he or she will have an autism spectrum disorder. Autism spectrum disorders may represent the most extreme outcome of the genes, but it may be just one of several possibilities, many of which are strengths. It is generally believed, moreover, that autism is caused by both genetic and (unknown) environmental factors that occur together. Research investigating both types of factors is currently underway.

How about the genetics of Asperger syndrome? Most of the research just summarized was conducted on people with autism. However, there are some hints that the information will also apply to Asperger syndrome. Several researchers have found that, when families have more than one child with an autism spectrum disorder, there is substantial variation between the children in terms both of how severely affected they are and of what specific diagnosis they carry. Sometimes a family with an autistic child will have a second child who has Asperger syndrome, and the converse is equally true. In the twin studies discussed above, the first twin always had autism, but occasionally the affected co-twin had Asperger syndrome or PDDNOS instead of autism. In other words, what runs in families is broader than just autism. This suggests that the same genetic mechanisms causing autism also cause Asperger syndrome and PDDNOS.

What about [Fill in the Blank]?: Other Possible Causes

Over the years, a number of other causes of autism have been suggested. There is some evidence, although it is controversial, that infections during pregnancy or in the first years of life may contribute to the development of autism in a very small number of children. For example, studies in the 1960s and '70s found that approximately 10% of children exposed to the rubella virus *in utero* developed autism. Other studies found that infections with the herpes simplex virus, which can cause brain swelling and brain damage, can in very rare cases lead to autism in a previously healthy person.

More recently, the late Dr. Reed Warren, an internationally renowned immunologist from Utah, speculated that some cases of autism might result from an inherited immune system deficiency that makes children more susceptible to viral or bacterial infections. Unable to clear the organism quickly, the fetus or infant is at increased risk that the infection might damage the brain directly. Another possible mechanism that Dr. Warren proposed was that early infections might trigger an *autoimmune response*, in which the body's immune system turns on itself and attacks its own parts as if they were foreign invaders (like viruses). It is thought, for example, that a similar breakdown of the immune system's "self-recognition" mechanisms leads to other autoimmune illnesses, such as diabetes. In diabetes, for example, the immune system is triggered by an infection, but instead of just fighting the virus or bacterium, it attacks the body's own pancreas, killing the cells that produce insulin. The lack of insulin then causes the symptoms of diabetes. Dr. Warren proposed that some autistic children might undergo such an autoimmune process, but that the organ of the body attacked by the immune system in the case of autism is the brain rather than the pancreas. A few studies have found evidence of antibodies (immune proteins usually produced to combat infections) that "recognized" brain cells as "foreign" in some children with autism spectrum disorders. One further prediction of the autoimmunity theory is that children with autism should have a higher rate of other autoimmune illnesses, such as asthma, allergies, arthritis, diabetes, multiple sclerosis, and the like. Some studies have indeed found an elevated rate of some of these difficulties in both children with autism spectrum disorders and their family members.

You may have read newspaper stories or heard other media accounts linking vaccinations and autism spectrum disorders. In 1998, Dr. Andrew Wakefield, a British doctor specializing in diseases of the gastrointestinal system, created quite a stir when he and his colleagues suggested that the measles–mumps–rubella (MMR) vaccine might contribute to both chronic bowel problems and autism in some children. He described 12 children who had both bowel problems and autism that started in some (but not all) cases shortly after the child received the MMR vaccine. Dr. Wakefield hypothesized that the vaccine caused the bowel problems, which in turn led to decreased absorption of essential vitamins and nutrients, causing brain development anomalies that resulted in autism and other developmental problems. Another possible mechanism through which the vaccine could cause autism is related to the autoimmunity theory, in which a viral infection turns on the immune system, which for some reason malfunctions and begins attacking parts of the body instead of (or in addition to) the virus. It is possible that the critical exposure to a virus that causes this devastating chain reaction occurs when the child is vaccinated.

The suggestion that vaccines may be related to the development of autism spectrum disorders has been taken very seriously by a number of government agencies, as the public health implications are potentially enormous. Many medical research centers around the world are currently being funded to explore whether vaccinations can, in some cases, cause autism spectrum disorders. Preliminary results suggest that this is rarely the case, however. First, in a later study, Dr. Wakefield himself reported failure to find any evidence of measles virus in the bowels of the affected children, calling into question the mechanism through which the vaccine could lead to autism. Second, a large study identified all cases of autism spectrum disorders born in London from 1979 to the present. The researchers compared the rates of autism before and after the MMR vaccine was introduced in England in 1988 and did not find any differences. Additionally, they compared children vaccinated before 18 months of age to those vaccinated after this age or never vaccinated and again did not find any differences. They also showed that the rates of vaccination were no different in children with autism spectrum disorders and those without it. Finally, they showed that the first signs of autism reported by parents were not more likely to occur in the time period just following vaccination than during other time periods. Thus, it appears that if measles or other vaccines cause autism spectrum disorders, it is a very rare occurrence. However, many research teams are currently studying this topic, and we hope to have a definite answer shortly.

Finally, a number of pregnancy, labor, and delivery complications have been noted in the histories of children who later turn out to have autism spectrum disorders, such as maternal bleeding during pregnancy, high blood pressure in the mother leading to toxemia, prematurity, and oxygen deprivation during or shortly after birth. What several studies have shown, however, is that these complications are found not only in children with autism, but also in children with other disorders, including cerebral palsy, mental retardation, speech–language disorders, and learning disabilities. Therefore, it appears that obstetrical complications probably cause general differences in brain development, but do not specifically cause autism spectrum disorders.

It has also been suggested that such complications are not *causes* of autism but *consequences* of it. This interesting hypothesis speculates that obstetric problems may occur in pregnancies in which something has already gone wrong with fetal development. Evidence for this comes from children with genetic disorders like Down syndrome, whose mothers have higher than average rates of pregnancy and delivery complications. Down syndrome is determined at the moment of conception. Therefore, there is something different about the growing baby long before the obstetrical complications take place. Some scientists have wondered if a similar scenario could account for the slightly elevated rate of prenatal and birth difficulties seen in individuals with autism spectrum disorders. They reasoned that genetic factors, as discussed earlier in this chapter, act early in fetal development to in some way weaken or jeopardize the infant so that the pregnancy and delivery fail to progress normally. In other words, the complications follow, rather than lead to, the autism spectrum disorder.

Another theory relating obstetric events to autism spectrum disorders involves the use of the medication Pitocin to induce labor. When mothers have not gone into labor themselves and obstetricians feel that starting the birth is important, they administer Pitocin, which acts in the same manner as oxytocin, the natural chemical in women's bodies that stimulates labor. Oxytocin, in addition to causing uterine contractions, is very important to social behavior and attachment. It was speculated that if infants were exposed to a synthetic oxytocin, their bodies would decrease or stop production of oxytocin, leading to difficulty bonding with others. This is a common pattern in the body (known as a "negative feedback loop") ensuring that the levels of needed chemicals are neither too high nor too low. When the body senses that levels of a chemical are high, it signals the cells that produce the chemical to shut down. So, if a lot of Pitocin was circulating in the newborn infant's body, the theory speculates that the baby would stop making oxytocin, which would significantly interfere with his or her ability to bond with others. Interesting though this mechanism is, two recent studies have shown that the rate of Pitocin induction is no greater in children with autism than in other children. So, at this time, if you worry that labor induction or a difficult birth caused your child's autism spectrum disorder, most evidence suggests that you can put these fears to rest.

This chapter has included many hints and leads about the causes of autism spectrum disorders. Most scientists believe that there are a number, perhaps even dozens, of different ways for an individual to end up with autism or Asperger syndrome. So even when causes are found, each cause may apply only to a small group of children. New theories are generated every few months, some of which prove to be fruitful and others of which lead to dead ends. Parents often ask if they should have new medical tests performed as new theories about cause appear. Typically, doctors suggest waiting, because it will take time for a useful theory explaining autism to evolve, as research centers around the world tackle the question. The search for answers is a universal human need that affects both parents and scientists, so there is no doubt that the search for causes will continue and intensify in the future.

CHAPTER 4

Treatments for Asperger Syndrome and High-Functioning Autism

As Seth's parents heard the psychologist say "autism," they were engulfed in despair. "But," the psychologist continued, "there are some very good programs that have been developed to treat the exact kinds of problems Seth has." She handed them a slip of paper with a phone number written on it and encouraged them to call that very afternoon, saying, "They will take care of you and Seth." Seth enrolled in this special education preschool just for children with autism that fall. He stayed in this program for 2 years, until he was eligible for kindergarten. His parents asked his teachers what type of intervention he should have next, and were startled by their reply: "There are no specific schools for someone like Seth after this." While Seth had made rapid progress in preschool and could now talk very well, he still had many difficulties, and his parents knew that his need for treatment was far from over. Thus began their long search for therapies, programs, and classes that would help their bright, talkative, but socially inept son negotiate his course through life.

So Now What?

Obtaining a diagnosis may not be the most important product of your child's assessment. Even more critical could be what the diagnosis tells you about how to help your child. The rest of this book covers methods of treating and managing the difficulties associated with Asperger syndrome and high-functioning autism. This chapter presents an overview of the different treatment options available in many communities and, when known, their relative benefits and risks. As discussed in Chapter 1, the range of outcomes seen in adolescents and adults with autism spectrum disorders is wide. Some people improve a great deal and their difficulties become less apparent over time. They function fairly well in a variety of different roles and settings typical for their age—college student, employee, roommate, friend, neighbor—with few apparent impairments. In this chapter you'll learn which currently available treatments seem to maximize the likelihood of these best outcomes. We hope that as more children are diagnosed and treated early, more will function well in adolescence and adulthood—perhaps a lot more.

Very little research has been done on the effectiveness of the treatment approaches discussed in this chapter. Most was conducted with children who have a diagnosis of classical autism, especially those with more profound learning and language disabilities. In fact you may already be familiar with some of the treatments for children with classical autism, because they are more likely to be spotlighted by the media. In contrast, interventions for high-functioning autism spectrum disorders, especially Asperger syndrome, are not widely known, even among practitioners. We hope this chapter will bridge the gap and thus spare you the frustration of seeking out this information on your own, as parents have so often had to do in the past.

You will, however, probably have to do a good deal of the tracking down, setting up, and implementing of your child's therapies yourself. As you'll realize while reading this chapter, there is a fairly long list of interventions that may help your child. *Some* of these approaches will benefit *some* children, but very *few* (if any) will help *all* children. Even tried and true medical treatments like aspirin and antibiotics are not effective for everyone and may even be harmful to some people. Autism spectrum disorders and their treatments are no different. And only very rarely are the different treatments described in this chapter offered under one roof, by one agency, clinic, or therapist. This is the bad news that comes with the good news that your child has a *high-functioning* autism spectrum disorder. Unlike programs for children with moderate to severe autism, there are few comprehensive programs that address all the needs of the higher-functioning child. You will need to find a professional who can help you assess your child's specific skills and deficits and draw up an individualized treatment plan. You will become an expert in your child's abilities and disabilities, making decisions about which of the treatments to try, and educating teachers, service providers, and others about your child. You will become your child's best advocate. In some ways, this is less than ideal, as you are likely already experiencing a tremendous amount of stress while parenting your special child and supporting and raising a family. But there are no teachers, therapists, or agencies that can be available to your child 24 hours a day, 7 days a week, for the rest of his or her life. You are the consistent thread from one classroom to another, from one intervention to another, from one therapist to another, who manages all the details, remembers all the important facts, and knows what worked and what didn't. You will be heavily involved in teaching your child how to behave and respond in everyday situations when therapists or teachers are not present. You are a critical ingredient in your child's life. The rest of this chapter, and this book, will give you the resources, skills, and support to shoulder this role while minimizing the tremendous burden it can represent.

Naturally, your first question and fondest hope centers on whether there are any treatments that can *cure* autism spectrum disorders. Assertions that there are, which you may have heard, are very controversial, because documentable "cures" have been few and far between. If this seems like disheartening news, think of AS-HFA as similar to diabetes, asthma, and arthritis: there are treatments available that can help each of these conditions considerably, even if they don't result in a cure. There's a wealth of things you can do to live with the illness, help your child feel more comfortable at school and in social settings, and create a normal, healthy family atmosphere. One mother shares her story:

"We were devastated when Spencer was diagnosed with autism when he was 3. It seemed as if all our hopes and dreams for him evaporated in the couple of seconds it took for the doctor to tell us what was wrong. We didn't want to believe it at first, but the description of autism fit to a tee, from his constant repetition of dialogue from Disney videos to his trouble looking us in the eye. Eventually we had to accept that Spencer had high-functioning autism. So we both took a deep breath and vowed we'd find a cure.

Surely there was something we could do to reclaim a bright future for this little boy we loved so much. We thought our quest was over when we read one day on the Internet about an experimental procedure that required intravenous administration of specific medicines and often resulted, according to this website, in 'turn-arounds that are nothing short of miraculous.' When we then saw the same treatment profiled on a primetime TV news magazine, and the children shown no longer looked autistic, we decided we'd get Spencer that cure if we had to go to the ends of the earth. Well, we didn't have to go to the ends of the earth, but we did have to travel 2,000 miles, all the way to the East Coast. It cost a fortune— we had to take out a second mortgage on the house—but, like we said, no cost was too high. Within a couple of weeks of the treatment we definitely started to notice changes in Spencer. He started to look at other people more often and began talking more. But that was about it. Once a couple of months had passed, we both had to admit that Spencer still seemed to have autism. We're grateful for the improvements he made, and we haven't given up hope that research will turn up a true cure while it can still help Spencer. But we've decided to concentrate on what we can do to help our son make the best of who he is. And the future looks brighter than we could have guessed a year ago. Spencer may have to struggle with the challenge of autism for the rest of his life, but we know now how much he has going for him, and we're confident that things will get better and better as time goes on."

Treatment Options in the Preschool Years

If you have a preschool child who was diagnosed with AS-HFA re-cently, you have several treatment options. Some of these have re-ceived much media attention, and you may already be aware of them. What you probably don't know is whether they are as appropriate for your high-functioning child as for the more severely affected children depicted in media reports. Some professionals feel that they are, rea-soning that if the symptoms are less severe, the child's brain is less af-fected and therefore potentially more amenable to rewiring, reorgani-zation, and the formation of new neural connections important for appropriate social behavior and communication. Research, in fact, bears this out. Study after study finds that the children most likely to respond well to all forms of treatment are those who are less severely autistic and who have higher intelligence and language skills—like your child.

The opposing school of thought says that children who are bright, verbal, and relatively more interested in social interaction (again, perhaps like your child) benefit greatly from the social experiences and language stimulation provided by regular education and other less restrictive preschool programs. These children often have better imitation abilities than children with more severe autism and thus may benefit from the modeling of "normal" behavior and communication by typically developing classmates.

This debate embraces our feelings and opinions about the nature of autism, the compassionate and just way to treat people with disabilities, and issues of segregation and integration. You, as parents, will have your own opinions about these issues, which may differ from those of the doctors working with your child. What you should know as you choose treatment programs for your child is that multiple intermediate options, in addition to the two extremes, also exist. For example, some parents enroll their child in an intensive behavioral program, but then also have him or her attend the neighborhood school for a regular preschool class, perhaps with the assistance of an aide. Another option is to actually administer the intensive treatments in a regular preschool classroom, rather than at home or in a special education setting.

Depending on where you live, some of the following interventions may be more popular or more available than others. Currently, these approaches are the most widely accepted and most effective preschool interventions. More information on each of them, as well as other treatment options, can be found in the resource list in the Appendix. Table 4 also compares their features.

Applied Behavior Analysis

The applied behavior analysis (ABA) model for treating young children with autism was developed by a psychologist named Dr. Ivar Lovaas, a faculty member at the University of California at Los Angeles (UCLA), in the 1960s. The treatment program uses general principles of behavioral therapy to build the skills that children with autism lack, such as language, play, self-help, social, academic, and attentional skills. In addition, the program tries to minimize the unusual behaviors of children with au-

Table 4. Treatments for AS–HFA

Treatment	Ages	How and where delivered	Features	Strengths and weaknesses
Applied behavior analysis (ABA)	Preschool to adulthood	In the preschool years, often at home, by a trained professional team, 30–40 hours a week, ideally for 2 years; later, techniques used in school and other environments	Use of clear objectives that are measured in terms of observable and definable behaviors, specific techniques for achieving those objectives, and ongoing collection of data to assess the effectiveness of the intervention; techniques are based on principles of learning, such as operant conditioning	Costly, but allows many children with 2 years of intensive treatment to function well in regular school without special support
Treatment and Education of Autistic and related Communication-handicapped Children (TEACCH)	Preschool to adulthood	Mainly at school, with home supplementation possible, by teachers and parents; techniques easily generalized to work environment	Visual structure and organization of environment and learning materials using visual, mechanical, and memory strengths to teach language, imitation, social and cognitive skills; one-on-one or in groups	Often funded by public schools; outcome less well studied than ABA, but it improves behavior and learning and reduces parental stress, increasing confidence
Denver and Greenspan models	Preschool	At home and school	Emphasize play, positive social relationships, child-centered control of interactions, and sharing emotions with others; based on entering child's world and letting child control interactions	Stress fostering warmth, pleasure, and reciprocity in relationships much more than ABA or TEACCH; less well studied than ABA, but appear to be particularly effective in increasing social and emotional skills
Social skills groups	Preschool through adulthood	Therapist's office, clinic, or school, led by therapist or teacher	Development of conversational skills, body language, perspective taking, reading of others' emotions, regulating emotions, and social problem-solving skills such as dealing with being teased or left out	Teaches skills and provides practice with peers; provides tools that translate to home training; can be used through adulthood

Educational support	Preschool through college	School	Accommodations to and modifications of environment and academic goals	Negotiable with schools; adaptable to individual needs; in elementary through high school mandated by federal laws
Language-communication therapy	Preschool through adulthood	Group setting or pairs of children, provided by speech–language pathologist	Training in pragmatics of language: social communication, abstract or complex language concepts	Beneficial when social skills group is unavailable or when child has more communication problems
Functional behavior analysis	Preschool through adulthood	School, home, and other settings, by any adult in charge	Examination of function of disruptive or problem behaviors; provision of more appropriate ways to communicate	Reduces behavior problems and increases communication skills
Medication	All ages	Prescribed by a medical doctor, such as a child psychiatrist or neurologist; given usually daily by parents at home	Presumably alters levels of brain chemicals that are affecting child's behavior	May be helpful for attention or activity level problems, depression, anxiety, anger, but does not treat core symptoms of autism
Sensory integration therapy	Preschool, childhood	Office of an occupational therapist, possibly with home exercises provided	Decreases sensory sensitivities, develops coping skills and tolerance for new sensations	Little research to determine effectiveness
Individual psychotherapy	Adolescence, adulthood	Office of a psychotherapist, potentially with "trips" into community	Explores moods and emotional states; develops self-awareness and self-acceptance	Best for individuals with good insight; may not generalize to group settings; needs to be as directive and concrete as possible

tism spectrum disorders. The treatment is typically delivered in the child's home by a team of trained staff. Between 30 and 40 hours of treatment are provided weekly, making the ABA model the most intensive program for autism and related conditions. Since the time that Lovaas published his original study on the effectiveness of ABA for the treatment of autism, the field of ABA has grown tremendously, and the techniques that now are incorporated into the ABA treatment approach typically are much more varied than Lovaas originally used. The ABA intervention approach includes certain features that are particularly useful when designing and evaluating intervention programs. These are the use of clear objectives that are measured in terms of observable and definable behaviors, specific techniques for achieving those objectives, and ongoing collection of data to assess the effectiveness of the intervention. The ABA model is particularly sensitive to the function of behavior rather than the form that behavior takes, and in this way guides the intervention toward meaningful objectives. For example, challenging behaviors, such as aggression, are approached using what is referred to as a functional behavior analytic approach (you will hear more about this in later chapters). It is assumed that challenging behaviors are often a means of communicating needs and desires. This perspective allows for an analysis of the reasons why desirable or undesirable behaviors would be maintained, which can be especially useful when a child presents with challenging behavior. Furthermore, the ABA approach is sensitive to the issue of motivation and drive, key issues that affect the ability of a child with an autism spectrum disorder to learn.

One basic premise of the ABA model is that initially, many children with autism spectrum disorders do not benefit from group learning environments until they have acquired basic language, compliance, attentional, and imitation skills. Thus, teaching is initially done one-on-one and is highly individualized, with specific treatment goals chosen based on the child's abilities and challenges. Once the child has mastered basic communication, social, and attention skills, he or she is gradually introduced into a group learning situation. A member of the treatment team at first accompanies the child to the classroom to facilitate transfer of skills between the two settings. The goal is to eventually fade the aide, or "shadow," from the class, so the child is then fully integrated into the regular school program. Some children achieve this goal, whereas others may always need an aide or will continue to benefit from participation in a special education classroom.

After reluctantly giving up on a medical "cure," Spencer's parents heard about a promising educational program based on ABA principles from an acquaintance whose son also had autism. They were referred to a local psychologist trained in ABA methods, who did some testing with Spencer to determine his individual needs. After concluding that Spencer would likely benefit from ABA, the psychologist recommended that a home program consisting of approximately a dozen goals be set up. Since Spencer was high-functioning and already had some useful skills (talking in simple sentences, sitting in a chair and attending), the initial goals were primarily academic: identifying colors, shapes, numbers, and letters; stating the functions of objects; answering questions (What is your name? How old are you?); identifying environmental sounds; imitating two-step sequences; and drawing shapes. Therapists came into his home 7 hours a day, 5 days a week, to work with him, and Spencer progressed rapidly. Within only a few months, he had mastered all of his initial goals. Spencer's parents also noticed changes in his behavior: his eye contact was better, he talked in longer sentences, and he was more cooperative at home and in his church nursery school. This was particularly impressive to his parents, because none of these behaviors were being targeted specifically, but rather seemed to emerge on their own as Spencer and the therapists worked on the academics. His parents were now not so worried about Spencer's cognitive skills, but still noticed many social difficulties. They asked that this become a more explicit focus of Spencer's ABA program, so exercises were added to increase his pretend play, his ability to ask questions and make comments, and his ability to take turns and follow rules of simple games. Over the following year, Spencer continued to improve, so his ABA team decided that he was ready for some integration into a regular preschool to work on his skills with peers. He began attending 4 hours a week, with a shadow helping him. Time in the preschool was gradually increased to 15 hours. By the time he was 5, his parents felt ready to enroll Spencer in a regular kindergarten class without any special assistance. He still had a few quirks, but he seemed as bright and ready for kindergarten as any other child in their neighborhood. They finally breathed a sigh of relief when Spencer's kindergarten teacher told them what a delightful son they had. She commented that he was academically advanced and chuckled about his habit of asking every adult what their license plate number was.

Research has demonstrated that many children, especially those who are high-functioning, begin treatment early, and receive 2 years of this treatment, are able to enter and function well in typical first-grade classrooms, without special support. In addition, Lovaas's study found that the IQ scores of treated children were far higher than those of untreated autistic children. So it's no surprise that the ABA program is very popular in many areas. An obvious drawback, however, is the expense and effort of one-on-one treatment. Almost none of the children that Lovaas's team studied who had received only 10 hours a week or less of ABA model treatment achieved the same success as the kids who had 40 hours a week of treatment. This has made professionals and parents reluctant to shorten or condense the program for economy. It is unknown, however, whether 40 hours are needed for optimal outcome, and many professionals now recommend 25–30 hours rather than 40. Unfortunately, there have been no studies to clarify what is the optimal number of hours of treatment a child should receive. The decision of the number of hours delivered often is based on practical concerns, such as financial issues, as well as the child's rate of progress or response to treatment, and the child's need for rest and other family activities. Because of the intensity of the program, school systems may not have a traditional ABA program in place. If you and your doctors believe ABA is the appropriate intervention, you may have to work with your local school district to develop the program for your child. This could mean making personal and family sacrifices in the process.

Despite this significant issue, we believe this approach is a good choice for many preschool children, so discuss it with your doctor. Information about ABA providers in your region is usually available from your state's chapter of the Autism Society of America (call 1-800-328-8476 for the phone number of your local chapter). The national organization called FEAT (Families for Early Autism Treatment) also maintains a web page that lists ABA providers by state (*www.feat.org*). Or your community mental health center or the psychiatry department of local hospitals may be able to steer you to regional ABA providers.

TEACCH

A second treatment approach in wide use around the world is the <u>T</u>reatment and <u>E</u>ducation of <u>A</u>utistic and related <u>C</u>ommunication-handicapped <u>CH</u>ildren program, which has come to be known by its acronym, TEACCH. This treatment program was developed in the 1960s by Dr. Eric Schopler, a psychologist at the University of North Carolina. A cornerstone of the TEACCH educational approach is visual structure and organization of the environment and learning materials. As discussed in Chapter 2, many children with autism spectrum disorders have difficulty with abstract, language-based tasks and instructional techniques, but have relatively good visual–spatial capacities. The TEACCH program capitalizes on the visual, mechanical, and rote memory strengths of many AS-HFA children, using them to develop weaker skills, such as language, imitation, cognitive, and social skills. Together, teachers and parents design an individualized treatment plan for the child that will be implemented in both the classroom and the home.

TEACCH programs typically structure academic, social, communication, and imitation tasks for the child so that what is expected and how to complete it are visually apparent. Visual schedules, consisting of pictures and words that show daily events in order of occurrence, help the child anticipate what is to come or the work that needs to be done during a teaching session. The child can then, on his or her own, without teacher prompts, "predict the future." Many children with AS-HFA tantrum or become upset whenever something changes. They cling to the familiar, not necessarily because they enjoy what they are doing, but because they *know* what they are doing and *don't know* what comes next. Introduction of a picture schedule can significantly reduce anxiety, frustration, and tantrums, in addition to promoting more independent functioning. See the Appendix for information on how to order materials to be used in making visual schedules.

Seth's preschool teachers implemented a schedule for him after seeing how sensitive he was to changes in the classroom and how much he thrived on routines. If Seth had memorized what was coming next (for example, lunch immediately follows a trip to the bathroom and washing hands), he was eager to move on to the next activity. However, even minor deviations in the routine, such as staying indoors on a rainy day, elicited shrieks of dismay from Seth, followed by many minutes of lying on the floor, kicking at anyone who approached. His teachers decided to begin using a schedule for Seth, which showed in pictures each of the major events of his day (see Figure 2). When something wasn't going to take place as usual, they used the universal

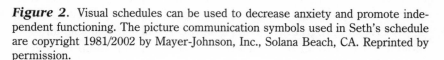

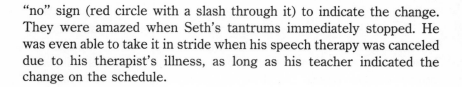

Figure 2. Visual schedules can be used to decrease anxiety and promote independent functioning. The picture communication symbols used in Seth's schedule are copyright 1981/2002 by Mayer-Johnson, Inc., Solana Beach, CA. Reprinted by permission.

"no" sign (red circle with a slash through it) to indicate the change. They were amazed when Seth's tantrums immediately stopped. He was even able to take it in stride when his speech therapy was canceled due to his therapist's illness, as long as his teacher indicated the change on the schedule.

Outcomes of children participating in TEACCH interventions have not been examined as closely as outcomes for children of ABA treatment. But studies have shown that children's learning and behavior improve after visual structure, organization, and teaching methods are introduced into classrooms. It has been found that many parents feel more competent and successful, and less depressed and stressed, after learning TEACCH principles and implementing them at home. TEACCH treatment is often offered in a school setting. Parents may choose to supplement classroom hours with home teaching, but the bulk of the treatment is delivered outside the home. Teaching is done in both one-on-one and group formats, but the number of hours of individual teaching is clearly less than in the ABA model. TEACCH also does not involve as many total hours of treatment as the ABA method. Many professionals believe that no one program will always work best for all children and that there will be an interaction between certain child characteristics and certain intervention program characteristics. Furthermore, many people choose to combine elements of the TEACCH model (such as visual schedules) with elements of the traditional ABA program. The approaches advocated by ABA and TEACCH can be integrated to best meet the needs of an individual child. You may want to explore, along with your doctor, whether the visual structuring approach of TEACCH may be useful for your child. Particularly if you choose not to go after an intensive ABA program and instead plan to avail yourself of resources provided by your school district, some structuring of the learning environment, in the ways suggested by the TEACCH model, may be helpful.

Other Preschool Possibilities

Several other treatment approaches have been gaining popularity for young children with autism spectrum disorders, including the Denver Treatment Model, developed by Dr. Sally Rogers at the University of Colorado Health Sciences Center, and the Greenspan model, developed by Dr. Stanley Greenspan of George Washington University Medical Center. These approaches emphasize play, positive social relationships, child-centered control of interactions, and sharing emotions with others. The importance of following the child's lead, "tempting" him or her to communicate and relate by entering the child's world, and allowing the child to exert control over interactions is stressed by these models. One goal of these therapies—a goal that is emphasized much more than in either the ABA or TEACCH models—is to foster warmth, pleasure, and reciprocity in relationships. These models also incorporate structured teaching sessions and behavioral and visual principles to address academic and other skills, and thus are somewhat more eclectic than either the ABA or TEACCH programs.

The Denver and Greenspan approaches have some research support for their effectiveness. At present, however, no studies have directly compared any of the four approaches just described. Thus, which programs have most benefit for which children is not certain. We recommend that you find the options available in your community, visit and observe the therapists or schools offering them, discuss them with your doctor, and weigh the costs and benefits to both your child and your family before making treatment decisions. Your local chapter of the Autism Society of America should maintain lists of programs, agencies, and providers and their treatment models. The doctor who diagnosed your child will probably also have a list of community treatment referrals available, as may your community mental health center or the psychiatry department of local hospitals.

Interventions for Preschool and Beyond

If the preschool program your child attends is intensive and comprehensive, then you may not have the time or the need for the following treatments until he or she is older. But what if you missed the preschool years and the interventions just discussed? What if your child was diagnosed after age 5? Or what if, like Seth's parents, you found a very effective preschool program and want to continue with some interventions upon entering grade school? All is not lost! A wide variety of helpful interventions are available for older children. As mentioned earlier, they may not be easy to find or readily offered to your child, but they *are* out there.

Some of these interventions use the same principles as the preschool programs just reviewed, so your child may still benefit from the use of behavioral or visual techniques, at a level appropriate for his or her age and intelligence. The two most common needs of children with high-functioning autism and Asperger syndrome are social skills training and educational assistance. There is a wide variety of different interventions for each, so we have devoted a separate chapter to each of these topics and will mention them only briefly here.

Treatment needs vary widely from child to child, but we have listed the following interventions roughly in order from most to least commonly needed.

Social Interventions

By now you certainly know that difficulties in the social realm are among the most prominent of the problems faced by your child. Naturally, therefore, they are an important domain for intervention. The many options for working on social behavior are discussed in more detail in Chapter 8. Social skills groups are one option that can be a particularly helpful resource. These groups explicitly focus on the social behaviors that other children seem to learn naturally. We can't take for granted that children with AS-HFA will absorb and imitate typical social behaviors just by being around others who perform them naturally (siblings, parents, peers). Social behavior is best taught in a social setting, and social skills groups provide that setting, along with the structure needed to teach these complex skills. Some common topics that such groups address include appropriate body language and eye contact, reading the emotions of others, and taking others' perspectives. Conversational skills and other behaviors important to interactions, such as introducing oneself, joining a group, giving compliments, negotiating, sharing, and taking turns, are a typical focus of social skills groups. Additionally, they usually address social problem-solving skills, such as handling teasing and being told "no," dealing with being left out, and regulating and expressing emotions in age-appropriate ways.

Your area may not have a group of this type exclusively for children with AS-HFA, but there may well be one for children with attentional or other behavior problems. The child or adolescent with AS-HFA often benefits from the opportunity to meet other kids with autism spectrum disorders who share similar interests, personality styles, temperaments, and challenges. But as long as the group addresses many of the issues listed above and you feel that there is a good fit between the therapeutic goals of the group and your child's needs, it is not necessary that all or even most of the participants have AS-HFA. You should also check with your school district, since often social skills groups are offered through schools.

There are also several things you can do around your home or community to improve your child's social behavior and provide opportunities to practice social skills:

- Write out "scripts" that help your child know what to do and say in certain social situations, such as answering the telephone or ordering food in a restaurant.
- Videotape your child having a conversation with someone and then watch it together, pointing out both things he or she did well and things that need improvement.
- Videotape others (perhaps siblings) to provide a model of age-appropriate conversation.
- Enroll your child in groups that revolve around his or her special interests so that he or she has an opportunity to meet like-minded others.
- Invite peers to the home to play and then carefully monitor the interactions and provide structure and support to help your child learn turn taking, sharing, compromising, and other skills.
- Set aside 15 minutes each day in which you converse with your child, uninterrupted by siblings, household chores, or the tele-

phone, about a prearranged set of topics (school, plans for the weekend, jokes). You might furnish the topics to your child beforehand or have them written down to encourage sticking to the topics and discourage drifting to your child's special interests. If needed, you might provide visual cues that encourage turn taking (perhaps an arrow that can be pointed toward the person whose turn it is to speak) and discourage verbosity (for example, a stop sign that can be held up to indicate that your child is going on too long).

These and many other techniques used in both clinic and home settings to improve social behavior are described in more detail in Chapter 8.

Educational Assistance

The second area of typical need is educational support. Despite average or better intelligence, many students with AS-HFA have difficulty in school or don't achieve at the level expected. They have difficulty organizing and regulating themselves in class and managing time, often resulting in failure to complete work during school and many extra hours of homework. They are often poorly organized and do not plan ahead, set appropriate goals and subgoals, and bring home what is needed to complete homework assignments. The child often is unable to discriminate major tasks from minor details and allocate time and energy accordingly. These problems with self-regulation, goal selection, and attention may result in spells of daydreaming or absorption in inner thoughts. Inflexibility and rigid problem-solving strategies also affect school performance. Finally, children with AS-HFA are often not motivated by the same kinds of rewards that other children are. They do not particularly care that their teachers or parents will be displeased if they leave work unfinished or get poor grades. They may have little intrinsic motivation to work on topics that aren't related to things that interest them. They may care little if they get detentions or have to stay in from recess. Therefore, it can be difficult to inspire the child with AS-HFA to do schoolwork, even when his or her intellectual abilities are high.

For these reasons, even children who are educated in regular classrooms or who receive only minimal special education assistance will likely need some classroom accommodations and modifications to succeed in school. There may also need to be some adjustment of academic goals, perhaps placing more or less emphasis on certain subjects, making work more or less challenging than that of classmates, or making schoolwork more directly functional. For example, you may want more emphasis placed on vocational and daily living skills than on a traditional academic curriculum. It may be necessary to start working on these skills earlier than would be typical for other children to promote your child's ability to live independently and function in a work setting as an adult. Year-round schools or academic summer programs are often helpful, because change is difficult for most children with AS-HFA and they can regress in behavior and academic skills over the long summer vacation.

In Chapter 7, we describe in detail the kinds of educational structure that appear most useful for students with Asperger syndrome and high-functioning autism. Many of the accommodations we suggest capitalize on your child's good visual skills and memory, using these strengths to make up for weaknesses in organization, planning, attention, and flexibility. The most essential part of educational programming is adapting the curriculum to your child's individual problems and unique abilities (more on this in Chapter 5 as well). At this point we will only say that, in addition to finding social skills training for your child, you will probably want to contact your school district to discuss the most appropriate ways to deliver educational support to your child.

Language-Communication Therapy

By definition, those with high-functioning autism and Asperger syndrome have relatively well-developed language abilities. They can speak fluently, in full sentences, with few or no grammatical errors. Yet they most likely exhibit some difficulty using language in a social context to exchange ideas and information with others. They usually have trouble with abstract or complex language concepts. When what we say isn't exactly what we mean (such as when we are sarcastic, joking, or using metaphors or other figures of speech), the child with AS-HFA may misunderstand. All these difficulties are collectively referred to as deficits in the "pragmatics" of language. There are rules that underlie conversation that the rest of us learn naturally and know implicitly. These include taking turns, providing enough information to be clear without being verbose, and contributing relevant information. We know how to choose appropriate topics, how to stay on a topic, and how to switch to a new subject. We know how to "read" other people and can adjust our communication to the needs of the person with whom we are speaking. If someone seems bored, we try to liven up our conversation or change topics. If someone seems confused, we try to figure out why and provide clarification. We speak differently to a child than to an authority figure or a peer. We understand how intonation or an accompanying facial expression can almost totally change the meaning of what we say. However, children with AS-HFA may not know these rules and often have to be taught them explicitly.

Much of this can be addressed in a good social skills group. (After all, how do we separate communication from social skills? The two go hand in hand.) But if no such group is available in your area or if the group does not address such conversational skills, you may want to explore whether some form of speech–language therapy would be helpful for your child. Ask around to find a speech–language pathologist with training in autism spectrum disorders. Find out whether he or she offers "pragmatic language" training or therapy in conversational skills. Often such therapy is offered in a group setting or with at least two children present. These skills are not well remediated in isolation, with just a therapist and your child present. Most children with Asperger syndrome or high-functioning autism perform well in such structured situations, where the demands are lower and the conversational partner is forgiving. These skills need to be practiced with other children, with the guidance of a knowledgeable therapist who can provide a supportive atmosphere and explicit feedback about the strengths and weaknesses of the child's communication style.

Another method proposed for treating some of the language needs of children with AS-HFA is the Fast ForWord program. This computerized intervention was originally developed for children with more general (nonautistic) language delays and language-based learning disabilities (for example, dyslexia), but it has become relatively popular in recent years for children with AS-HFA, despite limited research evidence to support its effectiveness with this population. The software runs "computer games" that work on language-related skills, such as discriminating different sounds in language. Children involved in this program must perform exercises on the computer daily for approximately an hour and a half, for several months (the duration of therapy varies according to the specific child's needs). The developers of this computer program have reported that children with pervasive developmental disorders (including high-functioning autism and Asperger syndrome) make significant gains in the ability to understand and use language as a result of this intervention. However, no one other than the program's developers has yet published research on Fast ForWord. Additionally, it targets aspects of communication (like speech-sound perception) that are not usually thought of as the most salient deficits in autism, so this therapy should be considered experimental at this time.

Behavioral Interventions

Children and adolescents with autism spectrum disorders can demonstrate some unusual and problematic behaviors that require specific management. Your child may at times have temper outbursts, possibly including being aggressive toward others or destroying things. When another teen called Josh, a 15-year-old with high-functioning autism, "fatso," he shoved his face into a water fountain, causing serious injury to the boy's nose. Or maybe your child is impulsive and distractible, shouting out in class, grabbing things from other people, or having trouble sitting and focusing on work. Perhaps your child is very rigid about routines, the order in which things are done, or where favorite objects are placed. One young boy named Mark insisted that boxes of cereal be eaten in order by weight—that is, if the Cheerios box weighed more than the Rice Krispies box, it had to be completely consumed before the next box of cereal could be opened. Mark also refused to eat food that was cut or broken—for example, he would spear an entire steak or burrito on his fork and then gnaw off bites. All of these issues can be dealt with by using *behavioral methods*, treatments that rely on principles of normal learning to teach more appropriate behavior. Behavioral strategies can be classified into two broad categories, those that modify behavior by changing what *precedes* the behavior and those that modify behavior by changing the *consequences* of the behavior.

Changing What Precedes the Behavior

The first approach can be thought of as a preventive approach. It is meant to stop behavior problems before they start, by changing things in the environment that are known to cause disruption, anxiety, or other stress to the child with AS-HFA. Many of the strategies described in Chapter 7 regarding classroom accommodations fall into this category. We encourage educators to teach the child using visual methods and to provide as much structure and organization as possible. This capitalization on the strengths and minimization of the weaknesses known to be associated with the autism spectrum disorders is just one example of the preventive approach to behavior management. Other examples include being sure that your child is well rested and not hungry, making sure that the side effects of medications are not causing behavior problems, and using visual schedules to increase predictability and consistency for your child. All these "interventions" are intended to decrease stress on your child and increase his or her feelings of control, and thus may be effective in reducing behavior problems.

Changing the Consequences of Behavior

The second strategy, providing specific consequences to mold appropriate behavior, derives from operant conditioning theory, made famous by Dr. B. F. Skinner. Most living things, from the simplest invertebrates to humans, from infants to adults, and from those with AS-HFA to those without, can change their behavior based on these learning principles. Specifically, if a behavior is *reinforced*, that is, followed by something good, then it increases in frequency, while if it is punished, ignored, or followed by any other negative outcome, then it decreases in frequency. We can use these principles to change the behavior of children with AS-HFA. If there are things we want to teach, we reinforce them. If there are behaviors that we want to go away, then we provide negative consequences for them. Most people with autism spectrum disorders learn well when provided with explicit rules. Reward systems can be set up that make it worth the child's while to follow the rules. Obviously, rewards that are effective incentives for children with AS-HFA are likely to be those linked with the child's particular area of intense interest, such as extra time looking up dragonflies on the Internet, a trip to the zoo exclusively to see the insect displays, and the like. But your child may appreciate other, more generic rewards, just like other kids, whether they are favorite dinners or special privileges such as staying up later than usual. Experiment, just like you would with your "typical" children. But before you come up with either rewards or punishments, be sure to explore preventive strategies, because some problem behaviors can be eliminated altogether through changes in the environment and other forms of structure. If this does not eliminate the problem or result in the desired behavior, then an operant approach may be successful.

Jenna is a young girl with high-functioning autism who had resisted sleeping alone since infancy. She would cry and tantrum when put down in her own bed, but would easily fall asleep in her parents' bed. They would then carry her back to her own bed. However, later in the night she would awaken, wander the house, line up favorite items, help herself to food from the refrigerator, and eventually climb back into her parents' bed to sleep the rest of the night. When her parents woke one night to find Jenna sitting up in between them with a library book and a pair of scissors, they decided to seek help. They first went to their doctor to explore whether there might be some physical reason, like seizures, that could be contributing to Jenna's night waking. After ruling this out, as well as making some changes in her diet (eliminating food and drinks with any caffeine and decreasing liquid intake in the evenings) that did not change her sleep, they were referred to a psychologist.

A behavioral program was set up that included clear rules for Jenna to follow and clear rewards for doing so. A bedtime routine was established that consisted of putting on pajamas, brushing teeth, using the toilet, reading two books, saying prayers, turning out the light, kisses and hugs, closing the door halfway, and then parents leaving the room. A photo of Jenna engaging in each of these steps was taken and placed in order on a piece of cardboard that was then taped next to her bed. The sentence JENNA, STAY IN YOUR BED was written on the bottom of the chart. Jenna, with her parents' help, made a list of all the things she would like to earn for staying in bed, including favorite snacks (which were withheld at other times of the day), small trinkets and toys, special activities with Mom and Dad (making cookies, going on a walk around the neighborhood, playing a game), access to favorite videos, and so forth. Each was written on a piece of paper and then put in a box covered with question marks.

Jenna was given a progressive schedule for earning these rewards, which she accessed by pulling a slip of paper from the "mystery" box. For the first week, she could earn a reward just by cooperatively following the beginning parts of the bedtime routine schedule. In the second week, she could earn a reward by staying in bed without crying for 1 minute; she was then permitted to sleep in her parents' bed as usual. This time was gradually lengthened and Jenna could earn the reward only by staying in bed for longer and longer periods of time. Eventually, she began to fall asleep while lying in her bed; then the required behavior for the reward became staying in bed throughout the night.

While it took many weeks for Jenna to reach the eventual goal, this procedure was successful in gradually shaping her sleep patterns so that they conformed with the behavior desired by her parents. Jenna greatly looked forward to her rewards and seemed to be highly motivated by the mystery involved in not knowing exactly what she would earn. Jenna's parents gradually lengthened the interval between the behavior and the rewards (for example, she needed to sleep in her own bed each night for a week to earn one) until Jenna seemed to have forgotten all about the rewards and had firmly established the new behavior.

The plan to help Jenna sleep in her own bed has several important ingredients to highlight. Her parents first explored *possible causes* of the problem, such as seizures and caffeine intake, and made environmental changes. Then they established a behavioral plan that had *clear, predictable rules* that were provided to Jenna in a *visual format*. They made sure that the *rewards were actually reinforcing* to Jenna by having her choose them. The requirements for reinforcement were at first set very low, so that Jenna experienced *immediate success*. There was a *gradual shaping of behavior* and a *gradual fading of rewards*, so that Jenna had to work harder over time to earn reinforcement, and expectations were slowly made more age-appropriate.

If necessary, negative consequences can be added to such a behavioral plan. Jenna's parents did not find it necessary to do this, but they could have added another component to the plan indicating what would happen if Jenna did not achieve the specified goal. For example, in addition to not earning the desired reward, she might have lost some small privilege if she got out of bed (5 minutes less television the next evening).

Methods like this can also be used to reduce obsessive or repetitive behavior. The key ingredients to all such plans include exploring contributing factors in the environment, setting up explicit rules and consequences, consistently adhering to them, and increasing demands in a stepwise fashion so that change is introduced gradually. Dr. Patricia Howlin, a British psychologist who has worked with people with autism spectrum disorders for many years, described using these principles to gradually decrease a young boy's obsession with "Thomas the Tank Engine" trains. A picture calendar was made that showed when access to the trains was allowed. Less popular "Thomas" activities were substituted for more preferred ones (such as reading a "Thomas" book rather than watching a video). Engaging in alternate activities was strongly rewarded as reinforcement for "Thomas"-related activities was withdrawn.

Sometimes it is not enough to simply provide consequences for behavior and expect it to change. If the behavior serves a very important purpose, then it may persist no matter how many rewards or punishments are introduced. Let's say, for example, that a child continually interrupts and yells out comments and repetitive questions during class. If the child needs more attention from her teacher and yelling and interrupting are powerful ways to obtain it, then the behavior will be very hard to change until an equally powerful alternative is given to the child to obtain the desired attention. If the child is given a hand gesture or written sign that she can use instead, and the teacher learns to consistently respond to the signal, then the interrupting behavior may go away without any need for a behavioral system of rewards and punishments. Likewise, if a child gets agitated and begins hitting himself during class, an examination of the function of the behavior may indicate that the child is trying to communicate that a task is too difficult. If an alternative way of expressing this frustration and desire to change activities is found (for example, giving the teacher a card with a picture of a stop sign on it), the self-hitting may stop abruptly. Problem behaviors can serve many functions; in addition to getting attention or escaping from an unpleasant task, they might indicate a need for help, a need to obtain a desired object, or boredom. Chapter 6 contains advice on puzzling through the possible messages your child is trying to convey with problematic behavior. Finding alternate ways to communicate these messages and ultimately to solve the problems behind them is at the heart of this type of behavioral intervention, called *functional behavior analysis*, also discussed further in Chapter 6. Psychologists and educators use a variety of assessment tools to discover the functions of behavior and then change them. If your child is having such problems, ask a behaviorally oriented therapist about such strategies.

Spotting and Heading Off Trouble

Another approach to managing difficult behavior is to learn the warning signs that indicate impending trouble and then distract, remove, or provide other incompatible activities for the behavior. Some children show clear signs that they are becoming agitated, aggressive, or anxious. They do not explode out of the blue, but gradually escalate, first appearing worried or nervous, then muttering under their breath, then pacing and flapping their hands, and finally having a full-blown outburst complete with lashing out at others, destroying things, and being verbally abusive. A plan can be set up whereby the child is removed from the threatening situation and taken to a safe place. This might be a room in which he or she can pace, talk, or rant privately; a place with a couch to lie on and soothing music; or a therapist or teacher who can guide the child through relaxation exercises (deep breathing, counting to 10, visualizing alternatives, and so on—see Chapter 8).

Self-Monitoring and Reinforcing for Teens and Adults

Finally, some individuals with high-functioning autism spectrum disorders, particularly adolescents and adults, can be taught to monitor their own behavior and reinforce themselves, thereby learning self-regulation and self-management techniques. Such systems are best set up by experienced clinicians. The essential ingredients are teaching the person to recognize the behavior that needs to be increased or decreased; training the person, often using videotapes, to reliably identify instances of occurrence or nonoccurrence of the behavior; and then regularly monitoring the behavior.

As an example, let's return to the interrupting behavior discussed above. A videotape of the child in the classroom could be made. Then the teacher or parent would sit down with the child and the videotape and point out when interrupting was occurring and when appropriate hand raising and other behaviors were present instead. The child would then be trained to reliably recognize the interrupting behavior. Once she was able to correctly say, "Yes, I was interrupting there" or "No, that was not interrupting" about 80% of the time when watching the video, she would begin the self-monitoring phase. An index card would be taped to her desk; on it would be two columns, one labeled "Interrupting" and the other "Not interrupting." A watch with a soft alarm would be provided that would go off every few minutes. Whenever the alarm sounded, the child would have to place a check mark in one column or the other. By so doing, she would become increasingly aware of the interrupting behavior.

This recognition and monitoring of the behavior, in and of itself, is sometimes enough to alter the problem. Often several of the approaches described in this section need to be used in tandem. Changes need to be made in the environment, rules and rewards need to be set, alternative behaviors must be taught, and then the child can learn to monitor the behavior herself.

Consulting a Behavioral Specialist

While the best behavioral management plans seem like little more than "common sense" to many parents, it is often wise to create and monitor such plans with the help of a behavioral specialist trained in such techniques. Small oversights can unintentionally throw off the whole system. Children may be resistant to the plan parents try to set up, so it can be helpful to have a third party negotiate the terms of the "contract." Gradual fading of the reinforcement system can be difficult to manage, and assistance in determining the most appropriate pace to decrease the rewards is often helpful. Determining whether punishment or negative consequences should be added is best left to a professional. It is ideal if data are collected to indicate how successful the program is, when goals should be changed or added, and when new methods should be tried. With professional assistance, behavioral programs can be highly effective in changing some of the behaviors of people with autism spectrum disorders and alleviating much individual and family distress.

Medication

The use of medications to treat people with AS-HFA has increased in recent years, due in part to increasing recognition of the neurological basis of the disorder. Research studies have shown that levels of certain brain chemicals (neurotransmitters) are different in people with autism, sometimes higher than they should be and sometimes lower. Although there are no medications that can "cure" autism, appropriate use of medication can often increase the quality of life for both the child and the family. Medications can improve the child's ability to benefit from other forms of treatment and relieve significant distress for the affected person and those around him or her. For example, appropriate medical management of hyperactivity can help a child focus better at school and thus enhance the positive effects of the educational help provided. Similarly, easing social anxiety or reducing negative feelings about the self through medication can permit someone with AS-HFA to participate in and benefit from a social skills group.

A wide range of medications have been used for autism spectrum disorders over the years. However, as yet no medication that alters the core social and communication deficits of AS-HFA has been found. The drugs that are commonly used with the AS-HFA population address noncore symptoms and comorbid conditions, such as attention and activity level problems, depression, anxiety, aggression, repetitive thoughts or behaviors, sleep difficulties, tics, and seizures. The most commonly prescribed medications for those with autism spectrum disorders are selective serotonin reuptake inhibitors (SSRIs) such as Prozac, Zoloft, and Paxil; stimulants such as Ritalin, Dexedrine, and Adderall; and newer "atypical" neuroleptics, such as Risperdal.

The SSRIs are thought to work by increasing levels of the neurotransmitter serotonin in the brain. They appear to help the irritability of people with AS-HFA, decrease repetitive behaviors in some individuals, and generally "take the edge off" or regulate the ups and downs of mood and behavior seen in AS-HFA.

Stimulants and Risperdal, in contrast, act primarily on a different neurotransmitter, called dopamine, and block its function or decrease its level in the brain. Stimulants are the treatment of choice for attention and activity level problems and appear to work as well with children with high-functioning autism and Asperger syndrome who have these disturbances as they do in children with attention deficit disorders alone. Risperdal is a medication first used for psychotic conditions, such as schizophrenia, but now thought to be useful for the aggression, explosive or unpredictable behavior, and repetitive thoughts and behaviors that are sometimes seen in individuals with AS-HFA.

In a study published in 1999 by the Yale autism research team, 70% of their large sample of individuals with high-functioning ASD had taken medication at some time in their lives. More than half of those in the study were prescribed two or more medications simultaneously. There were no differences in the types of medications used for high-functioning autism, Asperger syndrome, and PDDNOS. The most commonly prescribed medications differed with age; stimulants, generally used for target symptoms of hyperactivity and inattention, were most common in younger children, while mood stabilizers (antidepressants, including SSRIs) were more common in adolescents and adults. The authors of this study noted that the high use of stimulant medication, particularly at younger ages, might reflect initial, perhaps partial or inaccurate, diagnoses of ADHD that were given before the autism spectrum diagnosis was made (see also Chapter 2).

How effective are these medications in treating AS-HFA? To answer that question, we will digress a bit to explain the process by which we evaluate whether a therapy (any therapy—medical, behavioral, psychological) actually works. An obvious strategy would be to give people with AS-HFA a medication and test them beforehand and afterward to see what the effect was. But more careful examination points out a few problems with this approach. Perhaps the symptoms would have gotten better on their own (for example, as the child got older) and the improvement had nothing to do with the drug. For this reason, therapy studies must use a *control sample*, which is a group of individuals very similar to those given the treatment—they must have the same diagnosis, the same level of functioning, be of similar ages, and so on—who differ only in not receiving the treatment.

It is well known among doctors that many patients improve after being given a medically neutral or inactive substance (a disguised sugar pill or harmless salt solution), called a *placebo*, if they believe that it has therapeutic powers. This improvement is known as the *placebo effect* and is thought to reflect the powers of hope and positive thinking as well as the more general effects of receiving attention from a doctor. So it is important that medications tried with your child have been shown to be more effective than a placebo. Previous studies have demonstrated that about one-third of people show clear improvement from a placebo. So we would want to know that a specific drug helps more than 30% of those who try it. Otherwise, why not spare the expense and potential side effects of the drug and just use the sugar pill? This can be done in a research study in which the control group, rather than being untreated, is given a placebo instead.

The best studies include random assignment of individuals to the medication and placebo conditions and a lack of awareness on the parts of everyone involved in the study regarding which individuals are given which pill. Random assignment helps make sure that there are no consistent differences between the people getting placebo and those getting the medication that might account for differences in response. For example, if the first people to indicate interest in the study were assigned to the medication group, they might be more motivated to follow the requirements of the study or more hopeful of improvement, which could bias the results of the study. Conversely, if the first people to contact the researchers were those with the most severe symptoms and they were then assigned to the medication group, they might improve less because of their greater severity, again biasing the results. This is why assigning people to groups through a flip of a coin or other random procedure is so important. The second feature is that no one—not the parents, not the individual, and not even the doctor—knows who is getting the drug and who is receiving the placebo. This kind of investigation is called a *double-blind study* and again serves to minimize any biases that might be introduced (probably unintentionally) into the study.

A few double-blind, randomized studies have demonstrated that both some of the SSRIs and the atypical neuroleptic Risperdal are indeed more helpful than placebo for people with autism spectrum disorders. In no case, however, did these medications "cure" or even significantly improve the core symptoms of autism, such as social difficulties or communication oddities. Typically, they addressed other problems, such as severe aggression, compulsive behaviors, or mood problems. This research is still in its infancy, and not enough studies have been done to be able to tell which individual characteristics predict the best success. For example, does the medication work best with a particular age individual or with people with certain specific problems? And most medications carry some chance of side effects, so it is important to weigh risks, inconveniences, and financial costs carefully against the improvement that might be seen. Currently, double-blind, placebo-controlled, randomized studies suggest that medications can ease certain symptoms and thereby improve the quality of life for people with AS-HFA, but cannot alter the basic features of autism spectrum disorders.

Sensory Integration Therapy

Some children with high-functioning autism and Asperger syndrome are overly sensitive to and easily overwhelmed by everyday sensations, such as certain sounds, tastes, textures, or smells, or by being touched. Their distress when encountering these sensations can be very intense. Parents sometimes describe the phenomenon as "sensory overload." One young woman said that when she was bombarded by unwanted sounds, smells, and sights, her body would "shut down." She described feeling completely detached, almost as if her body belonged to someone else or was a piece of furniture. One boy with Asperger syndrome was so sensitive to smells that his mother called doctors in advance of his appointments to remind them not to wear perfume or scented antiperspirant. During one visit, he told his doctor pointedly that she had bad breath and threatened to leave unless she gargled with mouthwash. Many children with AS-HFA find loud noises intolerable and will cover their ears when exposed to them. Some even have difficulty with noises that are not loud and don't bother others, such as the hum of an air conditioner or the sound of a baby crying. Other children have the opposite problem: they seem to crave certain sensations and will go out of their way (often inappropriately) to seek the sensations. For example, one young child diagnosed with high-functioning autism loved the texture of pantyhose. He could tell if a woman was wearing them from long distances and would do everything in his power to get near enough to feel them. A girl with autism loved to press her chin into the soft inner surface of people's elbows. Dr. Temple Grandin, the famed animal scientist with autism, craved the feeling of deep pressure; as a child, she would lie under couch cushions to create this sensation and later went on to develop her patented "squeeze machine" for the same purpose.

Sensory integration (SI) is the name of the process by which incoming sensations are interpreted, connected, and organized, something that is necessary for a child to feel safe and comfortable and able to function effectively in the environment. When a child is not able to make sense of sensory experiences, his or her behavior and learning may be profoundly affected, according to a theory by Dr. Jean Ayres. She suggests that the unusual behaviors just described are due to sensory integrative dysfunction. Dr. Ayres noted that not only children with autism spectrum disorders, but also those with learning disabilities, cerebral palsy, and genetic syndromes, may suffer from sensory integrative dysfunction.

The goal of SI therapy is to decrease existing sensitivities, provide coping skills for remaining sensitivities, and increase tolerance for new sensations. This is done by exposing the child to a variety of sensory experiences through play and movement. The child is helped to explore many different materials and sensations. He or she is given some control over the experiences in therapy but is also guided through certain activities, such as swinging, light brushing, or deep pressure, that are thought to promote better organization and interpretation of sensory input. A child who is very cautious, for example, might be guided gently through jumping activities, whereas a child who is wild and uncontained might learn to crawl through a tunnel of small chairs to learn more about spatial boundaries. Children usually enjoy the therapy, because the treatment setting is filled with fun things to climb and move on, such as ramps, platforms, mats, trapeze, and tubes. Sensory integration therapy is usually delivered by an occupational therapist. It is important to find a professional who has training in the underlying theory, as well as the specific techniques, of this treatment model.

Despite frequent anecdotal accounts from both professionals and parents that SI therapy can improve behavior and functioning, there is little scientific validation for this technique as yet. In fact, some studies have shown that SI interventions are no better than other more traditional therapies, such as those reviewed above. Nevertheless, many parents and children themselves report a calming effect with SI approaches. You may want to try them out, but as with all treatments reviewed here and especially those for which there is little research support, be skeptical and carefully assess the benefits you see. Do others, especially those unaware of the treatment, notice any changes in your child's behavior? Are any benefits you notice above and beyond those your child might show following a good night of sleep or participation in some other preferred or calming activity (like watching a favorite video)? You may find it helpful to keep a chart of your child's behavior, something as simple as two columns on a piece of paper for each day, one containing information about sleep, diet, therapy, and special circumstances, and the other containing information about your child's behavior that day. In this way, you can keep track of any major changes and then examine their association with events in your child's life, including therapy. As always, financial cost introduces some limits. It is not possible to access every type of therapy for your child, nor desirable (from a time perspective) to do so. You will need to pick and choose among interventions and so be particularly careful in scrutinizing therapies whose effectiveness has yet to be established.

There are things other than SI therapy that may be useful in building your child's ability to organize and integrate experiences and body sensations. Movement and dance classes stress similar skills outside a therapeutic environment, as do individual sports and other fitness activities, such as martial arts training. You may want to consider some of these options as well.

Individual Psychotherapy

Traditional psychotherapy can help some, but in our opinion a limited number of, individuals with AS-HFA. Generally, individual psychotherapy involves discussion of emotions and gaining insight into behavior patterns or interpersonal issues. Since most AS-HFA children, adolescents, and even adults have limited self-awareness, do not naturally make social comparisons, and often show little insight into the nature and reasons for their difficulties, this form of psychotherapy is often not very helpful for them. Additionally, the realm in which the majority of problems arise for those with AS-HFA, social situations, are best dealt with in larger group formats, rather than in individual therapy sessions. One of the chief difficulties encountered in autism is the lack of automatic generalization, from one situation to another, from one interaction to another, from one setting to another, from one person to another. It is therefore unlikely that work done in a one-to-one setting with an understanding therapist will generalize to group social situations involving peers. Thus, group therapy (often in the form of social skills training) may be a better way to address the specific issues inherent in the autism spectrum disorders.

Under some circumstances, however, individual psychotherapy may be warranted, especially for the highest functioning adolescents and adults, who have gained some ability to understand their own and others' emotional states and behaviors. Individual psychotherapy may, in these limited circumstances, be helpful in dealing with the anxiety and depression that often accompany Asperger syndrome and high-functioning autism and the pain that may accompany the growing awareness of their differences from others. Counseling should still be highly structured and rather more directive and concrete than typical psychotherapy with nonautistic individuals. There should be a clear focus on specific problems, developing more effective methods to cope with them, and planning strategies to maximize the person's potential

103

and help him or her attain important life skills such as job-related social behaviors. The therapy may be highly directive and may even involve "field trips" into the community to encourage development of specific independent functioning skills (riding the bus, interviewing for a job, ordering food in a restaurant, and the like). In Chapter 8, we discuss one such approach, implicit didacticism, which was developed at the University of Washington, and is devoted to improving social behavior.

Stine Levy, an autism consultant in Indiana, is a pioneer in developing individual therapy approaches for people with AS-HFA. She suggests that visual structure, such as making lists on a wipe-board or piece of paper, is helpful even for higher functioning and older individuals with autism or Asperger syndrome. Since there is often a tendency to think in a black-and-white fashion, such lists can be divided into two columns: problems–solutions, pros–cons, realistic–unrealistic, strengths–weaknesses, helpful–unhelpful, and so on. Cognitive-behavioral therapy approaches, in which the person is helped to make explicit links between thoughts, feelings, and behavior, are often useful. Concretely associating specific situations with negative thoughts and feelings can help the person with AS-HFA gradually develop more insight into his or her behavior patterns and greater awareness of how his or her beliefs influence his or her feelings. This, in turn, can increase his or her sense of control over his or her emotional reactions and social experiences. We talk more about cognitive-behavioral therapy in Chapter 8.

Dietary Treatments

Some professionals have advocated the use of special diets, vitamin supplements, or both to manage some symptoms associated with autism spectrum disorders. In recent years, a theory has been formed that some cases of autism are caused by food allergies, specifically severe allergic reactions to gluten, a protein found in flour, and casein, a protein found in milk products, that irritate or damage the brain and lead to the unusual behaviors associated with the autism spectrum disorders. So far this hypothesis is based on clinical observations and parent reports rather than well-controlled scientific studies. As with understanding the potential risks and benefits associated with medications, future research investigations are very much needed. Some parents report improvement of their child's behavior when certain products are removed from their diet. When children are undergoing elimination diets (that is, diets that systematically remove one type of food at a time), it is not possible to have parents and children themselves be "blind" to what group they are in. However, it is perfectly possible to randomly assign children to diet or no diet groups and to have the scientists evaluating the children be blind to group assignment. This needs to be done before the effectiveness of these therapies can be known. It is always recommended that such diets be conducted in collaboration with a dietician or other medical professional knowledgeable about potential side effects or risks and who can ensure that proper nutritional needs are met.

Another form of dietary treatment for AS-HFA is vitamin supplements. Dr. Bernard Rimland, who was one of the first professionals to propose a biological cause for autism, has long been a supporter of so-called megavitamin therapy, which involves administering large doses (much larger than in a typical vitamin supplement) of vitamin B_6 and magnesium. These two vitamins are usually given in combination, because the mineral magnesium is necessary for proper absorption of vitamin B_6. Dimethylgylcine, or DMG, is another "natural substance" found in many health food stores reported to help autistic symptoms. Many parents report improvement in a wide variety of behaviors, including eye contact, social initiation, language, mood, and aggression, when their children are taking these supplements. A few studies have been conducted, some using double-blind or placebo-controlled methods, but the evidence of effectiveness is mixed. Almost all the studies had some significant limitations, such as examining very small numbers of children, not randomly assigning subjects to groups, or not using standardized methods of assessing change. We always recommend that megavitamin therapy be conducted with the collaboration of an experienced physician, because side effects of the vitamin treatments are possible, and doctors are not yet sure that the very high doses typically used are not toxic in some way.

Family Support

A final realm of treatment is the family. Relieving family distress should by no means be considered secondary or unimportant, although it falls at the end of this chapter. Many of the preceding treatments, if they are effective and help your child, will by extension help you and your family in general. To the extent that significant difficulties remain for members of the family, however, additional support may be necessary. Most urban areas have support or self-help groups for parents and families of people with AS-HFA. These are often associated with your state's local chapter of the Autism Society of America. In some areas, there are even regular meetings for families of children with high-functioning autism or Asperger syndrome, so that the topics of focus are specifically relevant for those with milder or higher functioning symptoms. If this is not available in your area, don't despair, because most support groups will still make a strong effort to have some of their meetings centered on higher-functioning individuals. You just may need to call ahead and get a schedule of topics to know when it will be most relevant for you to attend. Parents often find it useful to talk with other parents, who understand better than professionals what you are going through and who may have useful remedies for situations you find your family in. These support groups do indeed make it clear that you are not alone. Feelings of isolation at the time of diagnosis are almost universal among parents. Joining a support group will diminish those feelings considerably, as well as provide much constructive and practical assistance. Whether or not you attend regular meetings of such support groups, do contact your state autism society, an invaluable resource for community programs, books, conferences, and Internet sites.

You should also contact the government agency in your state that provides services to people with disabilities. There is usually a long eligibility process that takes into account the severity of symptoms, your child's functioning level and age, your family's resources (financial and otherwise), and the impact your child is having on your family system. If your child is found to be eligible under your state's rules, you may receive funding for a variety of different services (vocational training, residential care, preschool programs). Respite care is a service that provides trained paraprofessionals who can take care of your child for short periods of time, giving you and your family some needed time off. At its best, respite care is much the same as having a highly trained and trustworthy babysitter who is free. As your child gets older, your state agency for people with disabilities may also be able to provide vocational assistance, both in training your child for employment and in helping him or her find and keep a job. Additionally, there are a variety of assisted or semi-independent living situations that may be useful as your child ages into adulthood and you or the child desire new and more autonomous residential arrangements. We have more to say on this in Chapter 9.

Family and marital therapy can also be useful, especially if your family is experiencing significant stress related to the raising of your child. Parents may have significant anxiety or depression about their child's diagnosis or future, irrational guilt about having in some way caused the problem, anger and frustration about the availability of services, resentment about the effects of a difficult child on the family, and so forth. A skilled family or marital therapist can help you work through these feelings, learn to cope with the needs of your child, and still maintain some semblance of a life. If there are significant disagreements about discipline, other parenting issues, or treatment, a family therapist can be invaluable in constructively and adaptively addressing them, helping sort out the different choices, and disentangling personal or marital issues from the needs of your child with AS-HFA.

Parents as Treatment Managers

One of your biggest challenges as parents of a child with AS-HFA is bringing all the therapy options together into a cohesive treatment program that addresses your child's needs and promotes normal development in an integrated fashion. Your child may work on improving his or her social skills in an outpatient therapy group in a clinic, at school, at home, and in speech–language therapy. It is necessary that someone coordinate the different goals of each of these interventions, taking care that all involved are working toward a common set of needs and not at cross-purposes. Often this role falls to you.

Besides this day-to-day management, you will need to be aware of the changes in your child's and your family's needs over time. No treatment plan will be adequate forever. Some challenges will diminish with time and intervention; others may emerge as new developmental stages are reached and the skills needed to negotiate them change. It will likely be necessary to have your child reevaluated by a professional who knows both your child and autism spectrum disorders every few years to be sure that the treatment "package" continues to be useful.

The most difficult challenge of all, though, may be deciding which treatments to pursue in the first place. Most parents feel acute pressure to find the best treatment for their child. When you first hear the diagnosis of AS-HFA, you do not want to learn to live with it as a chronic condition. You want to *cure* it! You want back the child you expected, the child with a life ahead of him or her without the difficulties associated with AS-HFA. Often this quest involves trying emerging interventions that appear to show promise but have not yet been thoroughly researched. For some parents, the need to leave no stone unturned, to try *anything* that might be helpful, outweighs the potential risks and financial costs involved. But few of the interventions available, including the best-researched ones discussed in this chapter, have been studied adequately. And you can count on hearing about newly developed ones for which extreme claims of effectiveness are made. Typically, these interventions will not have been subjected to the kind of experimental research that provides information about what type of child benefits from the treatment, what particular symptoms of autism the treatment addresses, through what mechanism the intervention creates the changes it claims to make, and what "dose" of the therapy is required. You will have to ask the tough questions to determine the risk–benefit ratio of trying any such new therapy. For what age child does this treatment seem to work best? Does the child need to have language to benefit from the intervention? If so, how much? What kind of assessment is carried out before and after the treatment to determine the gains made? Be particularly suspicious of any treatment that claims to work equally well for all children with AS-HFA.

It may be even more helpful to talk with a professional who is familiar with autism spectrum disorders and the long history of their treatment before choosing new treatments for your child. Hearing about earlier "miracle cures" that turned out, once researched, to be ineffective may give you a different, wiser perspective. About a decade ago, for example, it was proposed that autism was primarily a motor disorder and that helping a child type on a keyboard was all that was needed to unlock his potential to communicate. This treatment was called "Facilitated Communication" and enjoyed much popularity in the early 1990s, bringing hope to many parents with severely autistic children. Later research demonstrated that what was typed was coming (unintentionally) from the therapist, rather than from the child with autism, *in every case.*

More recently, the digestive hormone secretin was touted as a miraculous "cure" for autism and received much attention on national news programs. Many children received intravenous infusions of secretin, without any evidence that it was effective other than the anecdotal media accounts. No evaluation of children before and after secretin treatment had been carried out to document the claims. Now five separate studies involving hundreds of children nationwide have shown definitively that children with autism show no more benefit from secretin than they do from intravenous infusions of saline (salt water, a placebo that has no therapeutic potential).

At the least, ineffective treatments are costly and delay the provision of effective treatments; in the worst-case scenarios, they may actually be harmful to your child. So be sure that all your questions are answered by someone you feel comfortable with and who has experience and expertise in the autism field. Be sure to check out local facilities and treatment programs, which are unlikely to have received media attention but may well be based on sound educational and therapeutic practices.

Throughout this book, we have emphasized the close relationship between high-functioning autism and Asperger syndrome. But you may be wondering whether the treatment needs of those with Asperger syndrome and high-functioning autism differ. No research has been conducted on this question yet, and as we've discussed, there is still general lack of agreement among professionals about how to actually tell Asperger syndrome from high-functioning autism and whether the two are really different conditions. If we find that there is a characteristic pattern of strengths and weaknesses that is typical of Asperger syndrome and different from high-functioning autism—for example, as Dr. Hans Asperger first described, those with Asperger syndrome having well-developed language, but being clumsy and less visually skilled—treatments that "capitalize" on the good visual strengths of autism would therefore probably be less helpful, if not ineffective, for someone with Asperger syndrome. In turn, those with Asperger syndrome might be particularly in need of certain therapies, such as physical and occupational therapy, to deal with clumsiness and delayed motor development, while not needing speech–language therapy. So the different supplementary therapies chosen might differ between Asperger syndrome and high-functioning autism. At this point, however, there is no research to support this division between Asperger syndrome and high-functioning autism, so in this chapter we have listed many options for you to consider. Whether the specific diagnosis is high-functioning autism or Asperger syndrome, your child's treatment needs are individual and will have to be chosen based on his or her specific strengths and weaknesses.

PART II

Living with Asperger Syndrome and High-Functioning Autism

CHAPTER 5

....

Channeling Your Child's Strengths
A Guiding Principle

B arbara and Eugene held hands as they drove home from Albert's
school, where their son was enrolled in first grade. Their hearts
felt heavy. Albert had been diagnosed with Asperger syndrome
during the summer, and now his teacher was reporting that he was having a very difficult time with both peers and adults in school. He wasn't
interested in playing with the other children, and he often refused to
follow the rules. Despite being very intelligent, he rarely did his work,
preferring to draw pictures of his favorite computer game characters. If
this pattern continued, he might not be promoted to second grade.

As the car pulled into the driveway, Albert raced from the house in
his stocking feet to embrace his parents and tell them about his most
recent achievement in his favorite computer game. Eugene looked at
his son's smiling face, felt the tenderness in his hug, and experienced
the now-familiar pain of knowing that others couldn't see how truly
wonderful his child was. How could he and Barbara help their son take
his enthusiasm and passion to school with him? How could they teach
Albert to apply the skills that had made him a neighborhood legend at
computer games to math, classroom rules, and friends?

Janice gasped in delight as she opened the wrinkled paper bag that
12-year-old Sameer had just handed her. Sameer rarely commented on
her likes and dislikes or on their interactions during their therapy ses-

sions, but obviously he had noticed the type of pen she used, remembered the single occasion she had mentioned her music tastes, and registered which snacks she occasionally left sitting on her desk. There in the bag, which he had taped closed and labeled "JA" in black marker, were her favorite model of pen, filled with ink in her favorite color; a bag of her favorite type of potato chip; and a homemade CD containing her favorite song—recorded 50 times. Sameer's naturally prodigious memory had helped him show Janice how important their relationship was to him, and Janice could see from his beaming face as she thanked him that this was a hugely satisfying accomplishment for this boy with Asperger syndrome.

For children like Albert and Sameer, everyday activities are often a big challenge. Normal, routine interactions with others can seem impossibly difficult. As parents, you can see your child's admirable, endearing qualities, but all too often the world seems blind to them. And because you spend a lot of time and energy helping your child meet the demands of the outside world, you too can end up focusing largely on your child's deficits and differences. This chapter offers you the opportunity to adopt a new mind-set, to begin thinking of your child's strengths first and his or her weaknesses second whenever you want to help your child navigate the waters of a world that can be difficult to understand. Chapters 6 through 9 offer a long list of specific strategies for helping your child succeed and enjoy life at home, at school, in the social arena, and, as the child matures, in the workplace and other adult settings. What underlies them all, however, is the simple principle that you can channel your child's unusual behaviors and ways of thinking into positive achievements.

Recognizing and capitalizing on your child's strengths, and helping others to do so too, can go a long way toward making up for his or her areas of difficulty. We've found, in fact, that asking yourself how you can take advantage of the true gifts associated with autism spectrum disorders, or how you can creatively use the unique ways of thinking or behaving associated with AS-HFA, tends to produce many more solutions than strategies that concentrate on attacking your child's weaknesses. By consistently calling attention to your child's ability to adapt in unique ways, you help others see your child's admirable qualities and also cement the positive bonds between parent and child. Perhaps most important, you help build your child's self-esteem. Success breeds success, and children with AS-HFA who are given opportunities to succeed tend to adapt to the non-AS-HFA world more quickly and completely than those who are taught to view life as one problem after another.

In Part I of this book we discussed how and why children with AS-HFA are different from typical children and what we do to try to overcome their problems. There is no question that trying to reduce the severity of deficits is an important aspect of treatment. Some children with AS-HFA are able to change and improve to a significant degree. But we urge all the parents we see not to stop there. You can tweak the environment too, in effect making it adapt to what your child has to offer. This is what living with AS-HFA is all about, and it is the guiding principle behind all the suggestions we make in the chapters to come.

This chapter describes six strengths commonly seen in children with high-functioning autism or Asperger syndrome and provides ideas for how to use them to help your child on a daily basis. You'll see them incorporated into our suggestions for living with AS-HFA at home, at school, with friends, in jobs, and in adult life in the following chapters, and we hope you'll focus on them whenever you have to come up with creative solutions on your own.

Though our understanding of AS-HFA is still in its infancy, we have enough information on long-term outcome to know that these children can live fruitful and happy lives. Dr. Temple Grandin, the extremely successful animal scientist with autism introduced earlier in the book, describes her achievements by stating, "I developed my talent area. Often, we put too much emphasis on the disabled area. You have to focus on the skills you are good at and figure out how to use them to work around your disability." Children who begin early to capitalize on their strengths are laying an important foundation for future success.

Inez is a 35-year-old woman with high-functioning autism. Every weekday she takes the bus to the campus of the prestigious university in her town and passes through the impressive, vaulted entrance of the campus library. She spends the day working in the archives department, locating old articles for students and organizing the library's collection. Inez has always been passionate about history, and this job gives her an opportunity to earn a living while keeping close to her intense interests. Her boss says she is the most efficient employee he has ever had, describing her knowledge of the university's archival collection as "remarkable."

Inez may never have gotten where she is today without the help of her parents. They realized that her interest in history, which often interfered with other aspects of her education, was not going to disappear and was an integral part of who she was. They resolved to stimulate, rather than discourage, her passion for history and make it applicable to the "real world" and future careers whenever they saw the potential to do so. In high school, they successfully lobbied her teachers to incorporate history into every class and many assignments. In this way, Inez broadened her focus a bit, learning not just about world history, but also about the history of science, the history of computers, and the history and evolution of different languages. They enrolled Inez in a history club, where she met adults with history-related careers (such as genealogy). Her parents even read some of the same books Inez was devouring so that they could chat about history at dinner each evening. When a job counselor mentioned the library archivist position to them, they recognized at once that this was a great opportunity for Inez to apply her enthusiasm in a productive way. After speaking with Inez, who was ecstatic about the prospect of working in an archives department, her parents spoke with her potential employer about her autism and both its special strengths and its limitations. He was open-minded about the idea of employing Inez, and he hired her. Although it took some time and effort for her employer and her parents to teach Inez about the rules of the workplace, she has flourished in the position and was recently named "Employee of the Month" in her department.

Inez is a good example of how the unique behaviors and special interests associated with AS-HFA, considered "symptoms" by the doctors who diagnosed your child, can instead be seen as "strengths" and can be used to help your child be successful in life. The six characteristics discussed in this chapter fall into two groups: *true strengths*, abilities that are beneficial in and of themselves; and *unique behaviors* that can be channeled into strengths with a little creativity and a shift of perspective. Your child is unlikely to demonstrate every strength we discuss or to be able to channel all unique behaviors into strengths, but through observation you should be able to determine which ones your own child possesses and which strategies will be most successful for him or her.

True Strengths and Natural Abilities

Many people with AS-HFA demonstrate a remarkable capacity for memorization, superior academic skills (particularly in reading and spelling), and/or strong visualization skills. These skills are valuable to school success and future career potential. Whether you have an autism spectrum disorder or not, it is useful to have a good memory, good reading and spelling skills, and highly developed visual–spatial abilities. Which can you see in your child?

Remarkable Memory

Other people often marvel at the remarkable memories, particularly for details and facts, of those with AS-HFA. In some cases, this memory can seem "photographic," enabling perfect recollection after only a single or brief exposure to the information. Other times, it is the sheer volume and precision of the memory that is so impressive.

Eight-year-old Robert recently astounded guests at his parents' dinner party when he told them, "The standard spacing of railroad tracks in the United States is based on the original spacing of wheels on an imperial Roman war chariot, which was 4 feet and 8 and one-half inches." Fascinated by the Greco-Roman War, Robert spent much of his free time devouring books on the subject rather than playing outside with the neighborhood kids and often regaled his parents at the dinner table with perfectly recalled details about what he had read. As his parents recognized his superior memory capacity, they encouraged him to use this skill in a functional manner whenever possible. They gave him a list of topics that other kids liked to talk about (the local professional basketball team, computer games, and so on), which he committed to memory and then used to converse more appropriately with his peers. They entered him in the town spelling bee, in which he placed second. And they encouraged his teachers to begin working on his multiplication tables, which he mastered in a matter of weeks. His parents were pleasantly surprised to find that Robert's prodigious memory was not limited to Greco-Roman War facts, but was in fact usable in a variety of other domains.

Superior Academic Skills

Besides having strong memories for facts and other information, many children with AS-HFA have stronger than average academic abilities, typically in one or two specific domains. Advanced vocabulary is one example. Learning and using new or sophisticated words comes easily to some children with AS-HFA, as we've seen in many examples throughout this book. Spelling is another common strength. And many children with AS-HFA can sound out or sight-read words far beyond their own grade level (although their actual understanding of what they are reading may be more consistent with their grade level or even lower).

One way to use this strength is to have your child tutor less capable peers in school. This can carry over to areas that may be more difficult for your child, such as social interaction, while also improving your child's self-esteem and potentially increasing interest in peers.

Norma had a hard time interacting with the other students in her sixth-grade class. They often teased her, and she frequently thought their interests were silly. However, she was an excellent student, particularly in English. She could sound out and spell any word, even those at the college level. The school psychologist suggested to her teacher that asking Norma to tutor kids who didn't read very well might be a good way to increase her self-esteem. Norma greatly enjoyed her work as a peer tutor. It not only showcased her talents and helped her feel valued by her peers, but also allowed her to connect socially in a predictable, structured, and comfortable way.

Visual Thinking

Many people with AS-HFA are what we call "visual thinkers," which gives them advanced skills in things like completing puzzles, reading maps, or quickly learning the layout of a building. In her book *Thinking in Pictures,* Dr. Temple Grandin describes translating words automatically into pictures. When someone speaks to her, their words are instantly transformed into a series of images that tell a visual story. She describes her thoughts as visual representations, rather than as the stream of words that make up thoughts for most verbal thinkers.

Much of our world was created *by* verbal thinkers *for* verbal thinkers. News programs and newspapers are in words. Instruction manuals usually rely on words, as do job listings. People communicate and interact predominantly with words. This can present some obstacles for people whose minds use a visually based system of thinking, but it also opens up possibilities to excel in ways difficult or impossible for verbal thinkers. Dr. Grandin, for example, describes how she can "test" cow-handling facilities by "operating them" in her mind, actually giving herself a "cow's eye view" and experiencing at firsthand what a cow would see walking through the facility. Verbal thinkers might be able to talk themselves through this type of experience, but they would miss important details.

By no means everyone with strong visualization skills has an autism spectrum disorder. Most artists, graphic designers, illustrators, architects, mathematicians, and engineers are visual thinkers. This style is simply a different way of processing information, not a deficit, and it opens up potential career niches not available to most verbal thinkers.

Ronnie, a college student with high-functioning autism, had known for a long time that he was a visual thinker. He had been using his visualization abilities to bolster his performance in school for most of his life. However, he never realized how much of an advantage visual thinking could be until he began the study of architecture. On his first project, he was surprised that many of his classmates were unable to detect design flaws until they constructed a mock-up model of the structure. Ronnie was able to think of a design and examine it closely in his mind. He could visualize the way it would look from different angles and the difficulties it might present for people using the space. He found that by the time he created a mock-up he had already worked out a viable design. This strength also helped him make social contacts. As his classmates became aware of his natural ability, many approached Ronnie to ask for his evaluation of their work.

You can also use your child's visual thinking style to teach concepts, explain rules, organize activities, or anticipate changes in routine. For example, the use of visual graphics or objects rather than verbal explanations or word problems may help your child more quickly grasp mathematical concepts. A fun way to practice math with your child is to use chocolate chips in addition or subtraction problems, allowing them to be eaten when your child provides a correct answer. The same principle could be used with pennies: you can allow your child to keep the pennies from correct solutions. Allowing your child to illustrate his work or to find pictures related to the topic she is writing about may enhance his or her motivation and learning.

For a visual thinker, pictures of things to be done along with pictures of the positive consequences for completing these tasks can be a strong motivator.

Annie's mother dreaded the daily struggle over homework. Every evening Annie protested doing her assignments because she preferred to sit and draw pictures. When her mother tried to talk to Annie about this, it seemed to "go in one ear and out the other." Considering Annie's strength in visualization (as evidenced by her superb drawing skills), her mother decided to ask Annie to help her make a pictorial after-school schedule: snack, homework, video, bedtime. Annie enjoyed making the schedule and seemed less resistant to follow it now that she understood what was expected and took ownership of developing it. If she completed all the items on the schedule on time, she could draw a star on a chart that accompanied the schedule. At the end of each week, five stars would be redeemable for a trip to the art supplies store to purchase a new marker or drawing pad. The visual reminder helped Annie remain aware that doing her homework each night would earn her the right to watch a video before bedtime. It also provided her with a long-range goal to help her maintain motivation throughout the week. Although Annie still preferred drawing to math, the adoption of a visual reminder system drastically cut down on the need for Annie's mother to nag and fight with her over homework.

Unique Behaviors
That Can Become Strengths

There are other characteristics associated with the high-functioning autism spectrum disorders that can similarly be used to your child's advantage. Sadly, however, you may be more used to hearing these characteristics identified as deficits. Problems that children with AS-HFA have in school and the social world are often related to their inflexibility, single-mindedness, and difficulty relating to peers. But there's another way to look at—and capitalize on—these behaviors and ways of thinking. With a little creativity and thoughtfulness, these too can become strengths.

Recognizing Order and Following Rules

People with AS-HFA often navigate the world by forming explicit "rules" or recognizing patterns about how things work, the ways people interact, and how events typically unfold. Parents are often amazed by their child's ability to analyze information and extract a set of patterns or rules by which something operates. One adolescent girl with AS-HFA commented that she noticed that one of the authors (G.D.) preferred clothing with horizontal stripes, whereas a coworker preferred clothing with vertical stripes. In fact, neither of us had consciously noticed that we had this preference, but when we mentally reviewed our wardrobes we had to admit that she was right. While we don't know exactly what facility enables people with AS-HFA to see certain patterns in behavior and conduct, we do know that this ability can compensate for the lack of natural intuition about social situations associated with AS-HFA. Rules, patterns, laws, and principles can help a person who lacks "common sense" about how to behave in certain situations feel comfortable and more sure of the appropriate course of action.

Denise is a young adult with Asperger syndrome who graduated from college and works as a medical transcriptionist in a hospital. In explaining her success, she divulged her "secret" of closely watching others to formulate rules of social behavior. Even when she was a child, she noted, she had observed peers for clues about appropriate conduct or comments. "I watched what they did or said in a certain situation and then memorized that rule in case it ever happened to me. And I was always so happy when someone would just *tell* me the rule! I remember being so relieved when my mother said that I should look at someone and give a wave if they said 'Hi' to me in the hall," Denise explained.

The same tendency can lead many children with high-functioning autism or Asperger syndrome to enthusiastically embrace existing rules and become great law-abiding citizens. The rules must, however, be clear, explicit, and consistent, or the AS-HFA child is likely to challenge their logic—possibly relentlessly. Albert, for example, couldn't help questioning why he and his classmates should be limited to walking in the hallways when running would get them where they were supposed to be faster. And why on earth should they share a toy with a peer when they were still having fun playing with it? To a child with AS-HFA, these communal rules and social niceties may seem arbitrary and counterintuitive unless the logic behind them is clearly explained.

The desire for rules and order can be used to enlist your child's help in chores around the home. Taking on household responsibilities can be difficult for all children, but if you match the task to your child's natural inclinations, it can be much easier.

Mark loved things to be in the "correct" place. As a young child, he would become very upset if the salt and pepper shakers were not placed in the middle of the kitchen table, neatly centered on a doily. As a teenager, he spent hours elaborately arranging his collections of rocks and bottle tops in categories according to rules his parents could never quite discern. Since he was so orderly, his parents thought he might be very good at mowing the lawn, but Mark hated the noise of the lawnmower and got very frustrated because the blades of grass didn't appear to be cut evenly. Instead, his parents asked him to help them clean their home office and organize their financial files. Once they generated the appropriate filing system, Mark undertook this task with gusto and performed as well as the best secretary. He later got a job at a local secondhand store, where he organized donated items by category for resale.

You can also use your child's inclination to follow rules to increase his or her social opportunities. Children with AS-HFA are likely to find social interactions that occur in rule-governed contexts more comfortable. A great example of social interaction in a rule-governed context is playing board games. Many board games not only follow a predictable routine, but rely on other strengths associated with autism spectrum disorders, such as memory and visual thinking. Examples include trivia games, spelling or word construction games, card games, and chess.

Passion and Conviction

Parents of children with high-functioning autism spectrum disorders often lament their child's single-mindedness about certain subjects or interests—usually to the detriment of necessities such as schoolwork, chores, and personal hygiene. But the very same tendency for focus makes these children diligent students of the subjects that intrigue them and very high achievers in those areas.

Darcy was diagnosed with PDDNOS in preschool, after her parents noticed she was exhibiting tendencies similar to those of her older brother with classic autism. Later her diagnosis was changed to Asperger syndrome. One of Darcy's special interests was computer games, which she enjoyed so much that she taught herself how to program her own games, earning her high status among kids in her neighborhood and at school. In junior high, she started a business making personalized screensavers for her parents' friends, earning her some much-desired pocket money. In her sophomore year of high school, Darcy volunteered in the computer science department of the large state university in her city, where she distinguished herself so much that she was offered a paying job the next summer. Darcy is now enrolled at the Massachusetts Institute of Technology (MIT), an accomplishment her parents never could have dreamed of when she was an isolated preschooler who spent all her time reciting dialogue from Disney videos.

Gene, who also has Asperger syndrome, is only in high school, but he's so passionate about chemistry that he's enrolled in college-level courses, where he excels and is a favored participant in class discussions. His professor was amazed at Gene's knowledge of the basic chemical compounds that make up everyday items, like cleanser and antiperspirant, information that he frequently shared with the class. The professor only became aware of Gene's diagnosis after mentioning this special skill to her neighbor, one of the authors of this book (S.O.). To Gene's professor, his knowledge was highly valued and practical, not a symptom of a disorder.

The same zeal for specific interests seems to instill in people with AS-HFA a strong conviction in their own beliefs. They can be virtually unwavering in the face of opposing ideas or arguments.

Laney was fascinated by recycling and the science of bioconservation. In her free time, she studied ways to reduce waste and increase use of recycled materials. When she first approached her junior high school principal about her ideas, he didn't really pay attention. But after she talked extensively with several teachers and paid a few more visits to the principal's office, he implemented some of the changes Laney had suggested. Her dedication and her passion had overcome the lack of interest of those around her and contributed to community improvement.

Whenever possible, incorporate your child's interests into school-related activities. By doing this often and broadly, you will maximize the likelihood that these interests will some day be channeled in a functional way that leads to a job or a career. For example, reading lessons might focus on topics that intrigue your child. English or writing assignments might be adapted to allow your child to write about his or her area of interest. Math word problems that incorporate the child's special interest can be devised. Catalogs of favored items (for example, sprinkler system parts) or menus from favorite restaurants can be used to teach your child money concepts. In social studies, your child can construct a timeline of important discoveries in the domain of her interest (for example, animals, computers, geography). Other examples of how to use special interests to motivate your child in the classroom are given in Chapter 7. How to find a good match between your child's interests and the workplace will be discussed in Chapter 9.

You can also use your child's special interest in a topic as a reward for completing chores, homework, or any other less preferred routine. An old adage of learning theory is "something of value should never be given freely." In other words, recognize what is reinforcing for and desirable to your child and make him or her work a bit for access to it. For example, allow your child to watch his favorite train video or read his plumbing catalog only *after* he's brushed his teeth and put on his pajamas. If your child loves using the computer, at school the teacher might make computer time contingent upon finishing a certain portion of work. But some caution needs to be exercised in restricting your child's access to his or her favorite topics or activities. It is very important to make goals realistic and rewards frequent. For some children, like Annie, who preferred drawing to doing her homework, making the reward contingent upon completion of a week's worth of homework might be sufficient. For younger children and those with a shorter attention span (or a greater dislike of the task at hand), rewards should be more frequent. It is easier to start with more frequent rewards and space them out as your child adjusts to the idea of working for access to his favorite items or activities.

Another way to use your child's zeal for a topic in a functional way is to find peers who share the interest. This can create new opportunities for social interaction and practicing peer relationship skills.

When Thomas, a teen with Asperger syndrome, was introduced to John, a typically developing boy a few years younger, the two hit it off immediately because both were fascinated by principles of engineering and their applications to environmental problems. The boys spent time together drawing up elaborate designs for machinery that would "save the world," and a genuine friendship blossomed. Because he enjoyed having an audience for his ideas, Thomas learned to become more flexible and less controlling in his interactions with John and thus avoided many of the pitfalls that had plagued his previous social relationships.

One of the best ways to find peers with common interests is to locate clubs or groups devoted to those interests. A child with Asperger syndrome who has expertise in astronomy or space travel might thrive in a science fiction club or a fan club for television shows dealing with the subject matter. In these settings, a well-developed memory and possession of a great store of knowledge about a particular topic is an asset and can earn social status. One child who took great interest in a fantasy-based card game had little desire to socially engage his classmates, and, in fact, this interest frequently interfered with his social interactions. On weekends, however, he looked forward to attending tournaments and playing against and interacting with other children who shared his interest. He described these tournaments as the only time when he felt he "really fit in." Another child, who was an avid reader, started his own book club. By having a prearranged topic of discussion, this group helped the child prepare for social interactions and provided him with assurance that he would know what to talk about. More on how to use your child's passionate interests in social situations appears in Chapter 8.

Comfort and Compatibility with Adults

Children with AS-HFA often have difficulty getting along with their peers, whose behavior they may find unpredictable or capricious.

Adults are usually more consistent and more accommodating than peers, so many youngsters with autism spectrum disorders prefer the company of adults. The fact that children with AS-HFA are sophisticated in their language use and interests makes adults enjoy their company as well.

Johan fastened his top button and smoothed down his hair. He smiled with excitement as he walked downstairs to meet his parents' friends who were coming over for dinner. Johan loved to talk to people, but he had difficulty interacting with the children at school. They often made jokes that were confusing to him, and sometimes they made fun of his conversation topics. But he always had a great time interacting with his parents' adult friends. They talked about more interesting things and they never made fun of him. His parents had noted this preference when he was younger, so they invited their friends over more often and encouraged Johan to participate. They found that even though these positive social interactions weren't with peers, each occasion seemed to increase Johan's comfort and interest in just being around others, both adults *and* children. His parents were delighted that his comfort with adults had translated into success with peers during a recent class trip to a nursing home. When students were asked to mingle with the elderly residents, many felt shy or uncertain about what to do. Johan didn't hesitate to introduce himself to the adults. The residents found him charming and were pleased to have his attention. Johan's classmates were astounded by the contrast with the hesitancy he showed during interactions with them. They saw a new side of Johan, and for the remainder of the visit many tagged along with him so that his adeptness with adults could cover for their own discomfort.

Identifying Your Child's Strengths

The six characteristics listed above are a good place to start in identifying your own child's potential strengths. But keep in mind that it's not always easy or simple to identify strengths. Nor is it easy to determine which behaviors that usually manifest themselves as weaknesses can be redirected to make them strengths. When your child's endless discussion of the detailed features of myriad video game characters is getting in the way of social interactions and family plans, it can be a challenge to recognize that this behavior is reflective of a great memory. Observe your child's behavior in a variety of contexts and consider the following questions:

- *What does your child enjoy?* When he has free time, what does he choose to do? What things does she ask you about? What things does he tell you about? What kinds of items does she ask you to buy? What subjects in school does your child enjoy the most? In what types of family activities does he or she have the most fun?
- *When is your child most successful?* Think about areas in which your child is currently doing well or has succeeded in the past. Are there particular subjects in school in which your child gets good grades? Does your child do well at spelling bees or memorizing math facts, but have trouble doing word problems or answering questions about what she's read? Does your child perform better in certain types of social settings than in others? Can he join a group of kids playing a board game, but not ride bikes with the neighborhood kids? Do adults often comment on how charming your child is and appear puzzled at his or her difficulties with peers?
- *What does your child not mind doing?* Also considering what your child least dislikes can be informative. Does your child willingly go to the dictionary to look up a word for you when you're reading the newspaper, but asks you to do the simplest arithmetic for him, such as "How many days are left in this month?" A child might refuse to help with mowing the lawn but not mind organizing the bric-a-brac in the living room or putting away the dishes.

It may be helpful to record your observations in a journal. Nothing elaborate is needed, simply a daily or weekly list of things that your child seemed to enjoy, tolerate, or succeed at and the settings in which the activities took place. Ask your child's teachers or care providers about the activities your child enjoys and excels in during class or after-school care. Compare the answers you get from others to your own ideas to obtain a broader picture of your child's behavior. See if a consistent picture emerges.

Depending on his or her age and abilities, your son or daughter may be able to participate in the process of identifying strengths. An open discussion with your child about his or her unique characteristics can build self-esteem (some additional resources for doing this are mentioned at the end of Chapter 8). One psychologist who frequently works with children with AS-HFA frames the task as creating an "operating manual" for the child. Explain to your child that you have decided to create such a manual to help the child better understand himself and to help others better understand him. Make a list of things you have noticed your child enjoys and excels at. Ask if your child agrees with these strengths and if she can think of any others. If she needs help, give some examples of possible strengths ("Are you good at reading? Do you like everything neat and in the right place? Can you tell if I'm going the wrong way to school?").

Finally, examine the observations you have made and look for patterns or themes. Use the list of strengths that we described as a guideline, but be open to other possibilities. Do the areas in which you've seen your child succeed have anything in common? Are there shared features in the types of activities your child prefers? During what kinds of activities does your child have the most fun? Do the things your child enjoys or is willing to do reflect strong memory, academic or visual skills, a desire for order and rules, passion for a topic, or a gravitation toward adult company?

Remember that every child is unique and that your child may show different strengths than the most common ones described in this chapter. Perhaps your daughter's verbal skills are extremely advanced, suggesting that explaining something verbally would work better than making a visual list for her. Maybe your son craves quiet and displays a calm, gentle nature that would make him an ideal candidate for a job working with animals. Be open to all possibilities. The main idea is to look for themes and commonalities among your child's preferences, inclinations, strengths, and passions and then to use them on a daily basis to inform all sorts of issues, from chores, discipline, and positive family relationships, to school and future jobs.

There are many practical reasons to take advantage of the unique abilities that are part and parcel of AS-HFA. Taking advantage of your child's natural abilities can make things easier for both you and your child. But again, the most important aspect of focusing on strengths may be the boost it can provide to your child's self-esteem. Many children with AS-HFA are painfully aware of their shortcomings. They work overtime at school, at home, and with therapists to try to overcome their difficulties. Often those who interact with these special and unique children fail to emphasize the many areas in which they excel.

Capitalizing on the things your child does well can help you feel good about yourself and your child. For your child, maintaining a focus on strengths and natural abilities can have long-term positive effects on motivation, self-esteem, and achievement. In the remaining chapters of this book, we give specific guidelines for how to use your child's strengths to overcome the difficulties often associated with autism spectrum disorders that arise at home, in school, in the workplace, and with others.

CHAPTER 6

Asperger Syndrome
and High–Functioning Autism at Home

Parenting a child with AS-HFA can be a challenging role. You already spend a lot of time and energy managing your child's treatment, coordinating your child's education, and serving as social coach in your child's friendships and extended-family relationships. At home, things should be easier. Often, however, they are not. The unique characteristics of children with AS-HFA can make their interactions with the immediate family and day-to-day household functioning just as challenging as school, social events, and other types of interchange with the outside world.

In this chapter we offer a set of parenting strategies for handling common challenging behaviors that occur in the home, from resistance to homework and chores, to protests against changes in routine, to difficulty accepting household rules. We'll provide disciplinary strategies that acknowledge that AS-HFA children are motivated differently from other kids and often learn appropriate behavior via alternate routes. Then we'll look at typically difficult times of the day, such as bedtime, and tell you how to establish routines that will ease transitions and help your child fit neatly into daily family life.

Of course, your child with AS-HFA is not the only member of your family who needs attention. Our work with parents has taught us that attending to the personal needs of everyone in the family—parents and siblings included—is essential to maintaining a healthy family attitude and providing the most supportive environment for your child with AS-HFA. So the second part of this chapter will offer ideas for attending to your other children's needs—and your own—while handling the demanding task of caring for a child with the unique characteristics of AS-HFA.

The Foundation: Consistency

As you've read throughout this book, and no doubt experienced in your own home, most children with AS-HFA have a difficult time when their world is not consistent, routine, and predictable. As parents, therefore, you should always make consistency a priority, in both your overall approach to parenting and through the establishment of family routines and schedules. Making things consistent, routine, and predictable at home will reduce your child's confusion and anxiety and help promote positive behavior. In turn, this will help turn your home into more of the haven that it should be for the whole family. As we discussed in Chapter 5, many children with high-functioning autism or Asperger syndrome have very strong memory and rule-following capabilities, which usually make them quite good at remembering and applying routines. This is a perfect opportunity to take advantage of your child's strengths on the home front.

Your efforts toward maintaining consistency in the home will be even more effective if your home rules and routines are the same as (or similar to) those established in other settings, such as the classroom. Taking on the task of working with teachers, babysitters, coaches, scout leaders, and other adults who may care for your child to make sure that all agree on a common set of rules and routines for your child to follow may seem daunting. But remember that, for a child with AS-HFA, figuring out the rules is an arduous challenge, so this "one fell swoop" approach can be invaluable. Even if it proves impractical to have everyone echo exactly the same rules of behavior, you can ensure that certain dictates serve as consistent principles, such as "no hitting" and "no leaving the room [or the building] without adult permission." Children who learn that any physical aggression, for example, will be followed by a swift response from the adult in charge will begin to understand some basic principles of behavior that apply to all settings. This, in turn, frees up energy for figuring out the social nuances and skills that can be so difficult for kids with AS-HFA to grasp on their own. You'll have to continue to help over time, communicating and working with teachers and service providers on a regular basis to remind everyone of the hierarchy of rules and of the framework for all routines.

Understanding Challenging Behavior

Some children with Asperger syndrome and high-functioning autism occasionally display challenging behaviors, such as hitting, screaming, throwing tantrums, repetitive arguing, or even self-injury (such as slapping their own face or biting their hand). For many parents, particularly when you are in the midst of a "spirited episode" with your child, these problem behaviors seem like an end in and of themselves. You may get caught up in the moment, focusing on the idea that your child's objective is to engage in the challenging behavior and your goal is to squelch it. Obviously, you do need to deal with the immediate problem. However, it is important to remember that challenging behavior is not just random and almost always has a function or purpose. Most often, the child is trying to communicate his or her needs and wishes to others. So, if you want to discourage the challenging behavior, you need to determine what your child is trying to convey through it. Once you understand what he or she is trying to tell you, you can provide alternatives for expressing that want or need that are healthier and more appropriate for the setting. This is the foundation of an approach to behavior management called "functional behavior analysis," first introduced in Chapter 4, which is a systematic way of analyzing the purposes of difficult behavior so as to devise strategies for reducing them. Here are the steps involved in functional behavior analysis, with suggestions for using them to help your child eliminate challenging behavior. Incidentally, these steps should be used whenever problem behaviors erupt, whether in the home, at school, in the workplace, or in the neighborhood. For the sake of consistency, the following steps should be used not only by parents, but also by teachers, therapists, and others who encounter the problem behavior in other settings.

Step 1: Try to Figure Out What Your Child Is Communicating with the Challenging Behavior

Common things that children try to tell us through their difficult behaviors include the following:

- Messages indicating that the child is confused and needs assistance:

  —"This is too difficult for me."

  —"This is confusing for me."

  —"I can't remember what I am supposed to do."

- Messages expressing a feeling:

  —"I'm hungry."

  —"I'm sick."

  —"I'm mad/sad/scared."

- Messages indicating that the child wants to escape from the current situation:

  —"I don't like this and want to quit."

  —"This situation is too stimulating for me."

  —"I need some personal space."

  —"When will I be done? How long will this go on?"

- Messages indicating that the child has a strong need for sameness, predictability, and routine:

  —"I feel overwhelmed by these new [or unstructured] activities."

  —"I expected things to be the same as before."

  —"I don't want to stop doing what I am doing [for example, favorite activity]."

  —"I'm not sure what happens next."

- Messages indicating that the child wants to access something or socially engage with someone but doesn't know how:

  —"Give me that [object, item, food]."

  —"I'm bored and want your attention."

  —"I want to play with you."

When your child behaves inappropriately, ask yourself if you can hear any of these messages in the behavior. As parents, you know your child better than anyone else and have perhaps experienced his or her problem behaviors across many different settings for many years. Instinctively, you may have a very good idea of what your child is trying to communicate. But it's not always that easy. Here are some suggestions to make the process of understanding the behavior's function easier. These suggestions are based on the actual process used by professionals trained in functional behavior analysis.

Pay attention to the circumstances and contexts in which these difficult behaviors occur. Note also the consequences that result from the behavior. Write these down over the course of a week and then look for consistencies and themes. It may be helpful to use a piece of paper divided into three columns to record your observations. In the left-hand column, describe the situation or context that immediately preceded the occurrence of the behavior. In the middle column, describe the behavior. In the right-hand column, record what followed the behavior. Here is an example:

Situation	Behavior	Consequence
Oct. 9, 7:30 P.M. I told Michael to turn off the TV and get ready for bed	Michael began crying and hitting the couch	I turned off the TV and dragged him kicking and fussing into his bedroom
Oct. 10, 6:30 P.M. dinnertime	Michael was making silly noises and faces	I asked him to leave the table
Oct. 10, 8:10 P.M. TV room, told Michael it was time for bed	Michael hit himself in the head and shouted "I hate going to bed"	I brought out his pajamas and prompted him to get dressed
Oct. 11, after school, Michael's sister had a friend over	Michael hit his sister and shoved her friend	His sister called me and I put him in time-out
Oct. 12, 6:00 P.M. sitting around the dinner table	Michael pinched his sister	His sister yelled "Stop it." Michael smiled. Dad asked Michael how far he got in his video game that day

After you've done this for several days, some clear themes may emerge. Are certain times of day or certain contexts often listed on the chart? Are the challenging behaviors that arise similar or different? You may notice that the behaviors themselves differ from day to day, but that the situations in which they arise are similar. Michael often has trouble at dinner, but also when his sister has a friend over. Are there any commonalities across those situations? Look at the list of five possibilities above and take some educated guesses about which is most plausible. Perhaps Michael needs more attention in these situations or maybe he wants to interact, but doesn't quite know how to. Michael also is easily upset when it is time to get ready for bed. Maybe he needs more help or doesn't want to make the transition away from his favorite pastime of watching TV. These hypotheses provide some good clues for how to change the behavior, which we will come to next.

If your child is mature enough, another method of making your guess is to check in with your child. Many children with AS-HFA will have a hard time articulating complex feelings on their own, but they may be willing and able to communicate their motivations if you facilitate it by providing them with a list or a multiple-choice question. For example, when asked why she refused to speak to one of her care providers, one adolescent with Asperger syndrome wouldn't give any clear responses. But when provided with a list of items (with some comical ones thrown in for good measure) and asked to rank the reasons she was giving the person the cold shoulder, she was able to make her motivations clear. This strategy enabled her therapist to understand the motivations for her behaviors and to collaborate in forming a plan to make interactions with the care provider more appealing.

Step 2: Consider How You Can Change the Situation So That Your Child Will Be Less Likely to Need to Express This Message in the First Place

Here are some examples of how a situation might be changed so that the need to communicate the messages listed above is reduced or eliminated altogether.

- If your child is expressing confusion or difficulty comprehending a situation, consider how you can make the situation easier to understand, more concrete, routine, or predictable. For example, you may need to simplify the task (break it into small steps or reduce the scope of expectations), repeat and simplify instructions, or offer visual supports such as written instructions or pictures to communicate what is expected.

• If your child is expressing a feeling or an unpleasant physiological state, try to remedy the situation. Feed him, take his temperature, get an appointment with your doctor to check for a disagreeable side effect from medication, or make sure he gets plenty of sleep.

• If your child is expressing that he or she is overwhelmed, overstimulated, and/or wants to escape a situation, consider avoiding this type of situation or reducing the amount of time spent in it whenever possible. If the situation is unavoidable, try to alter the most aversive aspects of the activity so that your child will find it more acceptable. Provide ample warning ahead of time and let your child know, using words or pictures, that a positive reward and/or break will be provided after the difficult situation ends.

Every Sunday morning, Amanda's complaining and repetitive talk began to crescendo as her family got into the car to head to church. Her parents knew that the length of the service and the crowd in the church were stressful for her. She had difficulty articulating her feelings on the subject, so she tended to act out to try to delay attending church. She also frequently asked to go to the bathroom during the service. Her parents made a rule that if she could make it through the service with two or fewer interruptions, they would stop by her favorite ice cream parlor on the way home. They even clipped out a picture of her favorite sundae so she could hold on to it during church to remind herself of her goal. After keeping a chart like the one described in Step 1 for two Sundays in a row, they also realized that Amanda's bathroom requests came just as the choir started singing. So the family began to sit in the back of the church, as far from the choir as possible, and allowed Amanda to wear earplugs when the singing began.

• If your child is having problems transitioning from one activity (typically a preferred activity) to another, make sure there are cues to indicate the upcoming transition (such as a picture or written schedule showing the order of activities). Provide plenty of advance warning (for example, by using a timer), and allow your child to have closure on the current activity (for example, by putting things away in a box, completing a computer game, and so on). Clarify what happens next and assist him or her with making the transition by walking your child through it.

After filling in the chart in Step 1 for a week, Michael's mother noticed that getting ready for bed was a particularly difficult time. She would ask him to stop watching TV and get ready for bed, even giving him a warning to allow him time to finish his favorite TV program. But, inevitably, he would then become very distressed, start engaging in repetitive talk, such as asking questions about the previous TV show, cry, and sometimes even be aggressive. He would calm down only if she stopped what she was doing and walked him through each of the steps needed to get ready for bed. It occurred to her that perhaps the frustration and distress he had shown earlier were his way of communicating that he needed help with his bedtime routine. She realized that, although each step of the routine, such as brushing his teeth and putting on his pajamas, in itself was not difficult for Michael, sequencing the steps and completing them independently was quite challenging for him. Because Michael was a proficient reader, she decided to make a chart outlining the series of steps required for the bedtime routine, and to encourage him to check off each step as he completed it. This not only helped him sequence and organize his behavior, but also gave him a sense of accomplishment.

• If your child is expressing a desire to engage socially with another child, be sure to provide ample opportunities for social activities, such as organized clubs. Notice whether other children are responding positively to your child's attempts to initiate interaction when they are appropriate. If your child is being ignored, consider ways in which you can facilitate more positive responses to your child (such as structuring a one-on-one play date, as illustrated in Chapter 8). If your child is trying to obtain a desired object, provide access to it whenever possible, or devise a plan whereby your child could earn access by completing other less favored activities first.

James loved to play on the computer, but he tended to ask to use it many times a day. If his parents didn't immediately respond by providing access to the computer, he would ask repetitively, sometimes hundreds of times in an hour, "When can I use it?" His parents truly thought they would be driven crazy! Following the "nothing of value should be given freely" adage (see Chapter 5), they decided to allow James to use the computer 10 times a day, but always following a less preferred activity, such as doing 10 minutes of homework, loading the dishwasher, or brushing his teeth. James was pleased to use the computer so often, and his demanding litany dropped in frequency.

Step 3: If the Message Must Be Communicated, Come Up with a Way in Which Your Child Can Communicate His or Her Needs or Wishes by Using a More Appropriate Behavior

If you can't eliminate the need for the message (as in Step 2), you need to help your child come up with more positive and acceptable ways of telling you what he or she needs to tell you. These include both appropriate verbal statements and more positive nonverbal ways to communicate the message and supplant the inappropriate behavior:

- Instead of screaming when confused by her homework, your child can be taught to raise her hand, ring a bell, turn sideways in her seat, or engage in some other nonverbal behavior that signals she needs help.
- Instead of biting his hand when asked to set the table, your child can learn to say, "I need help with this" or "This is too hard."
- Instead of hitting other people when she is distressed and wants to escape a situation, your daughter can say, "I don't like this."
- Instead of cursing and tearing up materials, your son can be taught to hold up a picture of a stop sign when he needs a break.

Whenever Eduardo became frustrated or bored during his homework, he would simply get up and leave the room and then resist coming back. His mother felt that he needed some breaks during homework time, but was worried that taking too much time off would mean he'd never finish his assignments. She gave him five index cards, each of which said, "Good for One 3-Minute Break," and told him that from now on all he had to do was say, "I need a break," and he would immediately get a 3-minute respite. Just knowing this "out" was available to him made Eduardo feel that his homework was more manageable. Although it took a great deal of practice and prompting for Eduardo to learn to request a break on his own, this strategy was eventually very successful in helping him meet his needs in an appropriate way. As time wore on, Eduardo's mother was able to reduce the number of break cards from five to two. She also progressively lengthened the time between when Eduardo requested the break and when he actually took it, saying "Okay, you can have a break after two [or three or six] more problems." In this way, she balanced the need to honor Eduardo's new, more appropriate communication with the necessity that he still get his homework done.

- Instead of crying and hitting furniture when asked to turn off the TV and get ready for bed, your child can say, "I want to finish this show before I put on my pajamas."
- Instead of touching another child as a way of initiating interaction, your child can learn to say, "May I play too?"

Step 4: Practice the New Way of Communicating

How to practice:

- Model for your child the more appropriate phrase or nonverbal signal he or she can use to communicate needs or desires.
- Have your child practice the new phrase or behavior before the situation in which it is likely to be needed takes place.
- During the situation, remind (prompt) your child to use the new phrase or behavior.

Vincent had a habit of shoving peers when they approached a toy he was playing with on the playground. His mother taught him to say, "I'm playing with this now. You can have it when I'm done." To help Vincent learn how to use this skill, she modeled the behavior, having Vincent approach her and try to touch a toy she was using. Next, she helped him do the same as she approached his toy. Then she accompanied him to the playground and observed him as he played near other children. When she saw a situation arising in which Vincent was likely to hit a peer, she reminded him to say the phrase they had practiced. When Vincent used the phrase, she made sure that the peer responded positively by ceasing his or her request for the toy. Finally, she talked to Vincent's teacher about using the same procedure in the classroom and at recess, so that they would all be addressing his inappropriate behavior consistently. The teacher agreed to practice using the phrase with Vincent at school and follow up by prompting him whenever necessary.

Step 5: Reward Your Child for Using the Strategy by Showing That It Gets His or Her Needs Met

You must make sure that the new communication strategy you've taught your child is as effective as the old one. If screaming or repetitive complaining is more effective than saying "I want to finish this video" or holding up a break card, your child will have little motivation to use the new strategy. Whenever possible, immediately reward your child for using the appropriate communication, first by praising him or her ("I'm glad you're using your new words") and then by "honoring the communication" and making sure the natural positive consequences occur:

- When your child requests help, immediately assist him or her.
- If your child asks to leave a situation, provide him or her with a break right away.
- If your child asks for your attention, stop what you're doing and provide some time, interest in, and engagement with him or her.

Your child will learn that these new, appropriate behaviors are just as effective or even more effective in meeting his or her needs than the challenging behaviors you are trying to reduce.

Step 6: Be Sure That the Challenging Behavior Is No Longer Effective in Getting Your Child's Needs Met

Leave your child no alternative for getting his or her needs met besides the new, appropriate method you've taught. Ignore the problem behavior whenever it occurs, but provide a prompt for the new communication. For example, if your child screams whenever she wants to avoid a situation, prompt her to use an appropriate phrase, but do not permit her to leave the situation while she is screaming.

Ivana's 11-year-old daughter, Michaela, had a habit of coming up to her siblings and classmates and touching them to get their attention. When she was younger, this type of behavior seemed appropriate, even affectionate. But now that she was approaching adolescence her mother was concerned that it would irritate peers and could lead to erroneous signals being sent to young boys. Ivana explained to Michaela why this behavior was not appropriate and taught her instead to say, "Hi, how's it going?" Ivana modeled and role-played this skill with Michaela, and she also talked to her other children about the strategy. She asked them to ignore Michaela if she touched them but to pay attention to her right away if she asked for their attention as she had been taught. This ensured simultaneously that Michaela's inappropriate skills would not be successful and that her new strategies would be rewarding.

The steps we've described are straightforward, but it is no easy task to switch your child from challenging behaviors to more appropriate means of attaining the same goals. It will be crucial for you to practice with your child and to ensure that appropriate strategies will be more reinforcing than those based on difficult or inappropriate behaviors. Some parents have lamented that when they try to alter these challenging behaviors, they seem to increase in frequency. Although it may seem counterintuitive, this is actually a good sign. When children find that their old, tried-and-true strategy isn't working, they often take a "twice as much, twice as hard" approach in a last-ditch effort to achieve their goals. This indicates that your child has realized the contingencies have changed. As long as you don't yield to this increased frequency and intensity of the problem behavior, change is probably imminent.

Strategies for Positive Discipline

As you may have experienced with your own child, many standard disciplinary methods don't work well with children who have autism spectrum disorders. Children with Asperger syndrome or high-functioning autism may not have good self-monitoring skills and may lack the ability to judge whether their behavior is appropriate. They may not pick up on cues that normally would signal that their behavior does not fit in, and they may not feel the embarrassment or shame that many children experience when they have behaved inappropriately. Nor are they always motivated by a desire to please their parents and other adults by behaving well.

When 10-year-old Ronald had his friends over, they would try to talk with Ronald's 14-year-old brother Peter to ask him about a video game that he had mastered. Peter had no interest in talking with his brother's friends, but because he had Asperger syndrome, he didn't know how to communicate his feelings appropriately and would simply shove Ronald and his friends out of the way. Peter's mother would then send Peter to his room for shoving his brother's friends, which actually rewarded his inappropriate behavior by providing him with the solitude he wanted.

Approaches like time out, which work well for a typically developing child, may fall short with your child with AS-HFA. In general, the following strategies are more useful for children with autism spectrum disorders:

1. Establish a set of concrete rules and be consistent in enforcing them.
2. Make sure your child knows what is expected of him by writing it down or even illustrating it with pictures. Tasks such as dressing, brushing teeth, and setting the table may need to be broken down into small steps. It may be helpful to visually describe these steps in either pictorial or written form. If your child responds best to pictures, use an instant camera to photograph each step needed to complete a task and post the photos in your child's room or another area of the house.
3. Describe your expectations in terms of what he is supposed to do, rather than what he is not supposed to do: "Keep your hands in your lap," rather than "Do not hit." This makes your commands more positive and prevents a pattern of nagging from forming. More practically, it cements in your child's mind a constructive alternative behavior for future use.
4. Establish a morning and an evening routine. If necessary, outline the routine in words or pictures (often called an "activity schedule"). Have clear boundaries for activities and signal their beginning and end by using timers or visual cues (for example, putting play materials away in a container). Provide concrete cues that an activity is coming to an end (for example, by saying "The timer is about to ring and then you need to turn off the computer").

5. Use preferred activities as rewards for completing nonpreferred activities (for example, "Once you have brushed your teeth, you can read your dinosaur book.")

6. Limit the time your child engages in nonproductive preoccupations by setting explicit rules. For example, your child may ask you three questions per evening about his favorite topic or may play on the computer for a specific amount of time each evening.

Strategies for Difficult Times of the Day

Mornings

Mornings are a particularly difficult time for most families. During this period of transition from sleeping to waking and from home to school, children are particularly vulnerable to problems with over- and under-arousal. For many children who find school a stressful experience, the morning is also a time of anticipatory distress and last-ditch escape maneuvers. A helpful strategy is to accomplish as much preparation as possible the night before so that morning moods are less likely to interfere with the routine. For example, by laying clothes out prior to bedtime and organizing school materials by the front door, you can eliminate two tasks from the morning routine.

It may be useful to experiment with different approaches to waking your child to ease the transition from sleep to alertness. See if your child reacts differently to being awakened by a person, a buzzer, or a radio. Some parents find it helpful to give "incremental" alarms, alerting their child that he or she will have to get up in 10 minutes and then warning him or her again 5 minutes before actually asking the child to get out of bed.

Mealtimes

Meals are also often a hard time for families with children with AS-HFA. Many such children are finicky eaters, and this can be compounded by special diets or sensitivities to certain consistencies and textures. Many parents begin to worry about a picky child's nutritional intake, and, as they make this a focus of attention, the child perceives this as an opportunity for control. In this circumstance, mealtimes can turn into a real power struggle. Many parents find it helpful to introduce new foods one food at a time and one bite at a time. For some children, an even slower pace might be appropriate. For example, you might proceed from tolerating new foods on the table or plate, to smelling the food, to touching the food with the fingers, touching the food to the lips, licking the food, placing it in the mouth, and finally swallowing it. Many children will not accept a new food until it has been introduced several times. Some research studies suggest that changes in eating habits may take 2 weeks or longer to be observable. So be patient and allow your child adequate time to adjust to something new.

If you are seriously concerned that your child's nutritional intake may be insufficient, there are several steps you can take. First, check your child's height and weight with your pediatrician. Is your child's growth in the reasonably appropriate range? If there is cause for concern, keep a log of what your child eats (be sure to get information about what he or she eats at school) and seek consultation with a nutritionist. It can be particularly important to receive nutritional consultation before implementing a special diet.

It is also essential to keep in mind that parents don't always get an accurate impression of what their child eats. The mother of Sandra, an 8-year-old girl with high-functioning autism, was under the impression that her daughter ate nothing but pretzels and cheese. After consulting with the doctor and finding out that her height and weight parameters were appropriate, she asked Sandra's teacher about her eating habits at school. She learned that Sandra regularly ate the entire school lunch, including vegetables and milk.

It is also helpful to keep meals consistent in terms of time of day. This helps your child know what to expect and allows meals to be incorporated into a regular routine. For some children, it may even be helpful to create a meal schedule or weekly menu to make mealtimes predictable. When it is time for a meal, serve your child's food with the rest of the family's food (assuming your family has the luxury of dining together each evening). If your child chooses not to eat when the rest of the family is at the table, make it clear that he or she may lose the opportunity to eat dinner that evening. This practice forces your child to adhere to a meal schedule, which helps a sometimes dysregulated body ease into a healthy eating pattern. It also capitalizes on your child's desire for rules. If a clear rule is set (for example, "Everyone eats together"), then it is more likely that your child will embrace it.

For children who tend to get up from the table, seating them against a wall can be helpful. This makes it slightly more difficult for them to wander and increases the chance that they will stay put. You can also use strategies such as those described above in the section "Understanding Challenging Behavior." What function does the wandering seem to serve? Would providing a few short breaks during dinner help? Would a timer that shows how much longer your child needs to sit help? Would it help to provide your child with conversation topics or scripts (see Chapter 8) for the dinner table, so that he or she would be able to interact more appropriately with family members? Would it help to provide your child with something to hold in his hand or squeeze under the table while he waits for the others to finish?

After-School Time

The period after school is another difficult transition time for many children with AS-HFA. There is no absolute rule regarding the most appropriate after-school activity; however, the principle of consistency applies here as well. As a parent, you are the expert on your child. Is school a taxing experience for your child, and does he or she require some "alone time" to decompress after the stressful day? Or does your energetic child need some time to run around and expend energy after being forced to sit in one place for so many hours? Is your child in an academic rhythm by the end of the school day, and should you "go with the flow" and do homework upon arrival at home? Think of what the most appropriate after-school activity is for your child, and keep it consistent from day to day.

Bedtime

Another challenging transition, bedtime can be a daunting endeavor, especially since studies have shown that autism is often associated with sleep difficulties. Bedtime routines, such as going to bed at the same time and engaging in the same prebedtime tasks, are helpful for all children, but especially for those with Asperger syndrome or high-functioning autism. Give your child plenty of advance warning and a countdown (30 minutes, 20 minutes, and so on) as bedtime approaches. To help your child wind down, make sure he or she engages in a quiet activity, like reading or playing a mellow game, before bedtime. Another strategy for ensuring "decompression" time is to spend some time with your child in his or her bedroom before you turn out the lights and expect him or her to go to sleep. If you sit with your child at bedtime, make sure that you are consistent in the amount of time you spend at the bedside. Be sure that your presence is not serving as stimulation that keeps your child awake. Some children find it reassuring to know that after they have fallen asleep, you will check on them.

Make sure that the bedroom is a pleasant place for your child. For some children, it is important to keep favorite belongings in the room. For others, it can be excessively distracting or overstimulating. Some children find the presence of soft light or music soothing, while others require complete darkness and absolute silence to fall asleep.

If you try these suggestions and still find that your child has sleep difficulties, you should consider checking with your pediatrician, who may suggest some medications to help your child with sleep. Chapter 4 contains some additional tips for creating behavioral and visual routines for bedtime.

Family Outings

For most family members, outings and vacations are fun and exciting. For the child with Asperger syndrome or high-functioning autism, however, family outings may mean a break in routine, unpredictability, unfamiliarity, and the need to deal with new people and places. For these reasons, they can be anxiety-provoking times for children with AS-HFA. Parents can minimize stress by planning in advance and letting the child know what it will be like. Try Carol Gray's Social Story approach, which involves showing your child a story consisting of pictures depicting the experience and words describing what will happen (Chapter 8 describes how to use this approach in detail). For a child who is apprehensive about a planned family outing to an amusement park, you might visit the amusement park's website and print out some images of the parking lot, the entrance gate, and some of the rides. Then you can write a simple story to accompany the pictures that helps your child know what to anticipate. Read the story together several times before your family actually ventures out to the park. There are many preprinted Social Stories available that are appropriate for both recreational and nonrecreational activities, such as visits to the doctor. The resource list in the Appendix contains information about ordering Social Stories.

It may be necessary to acclimate your child to a new experience slowly by gradually introducing it in small steps. After reviewing the new experience using visual cues such as a Social Story ahead of time, you may want to arrange a short visit to the new place or activity. Over time, your child is likely to feel more comfortable with the new activity, at which point you can lengthen your visit.

Chores and Household Responsibilities

Encouraging children to help around the home is a challenge for every parent, including those parenting children with AS-HFA. It is typical for children to dislike chores and to try their best to shirk these responsibilities in lieu of something more fun. To make chores more tolerable for a child with an autism spectrum disorder, embed them in a daily or weekly routine. This consistency will help your child know what needs to be done and prevent a chore from being an unwelcome surprise. Likewise, try to routinize the steps in the chore. Capitalizing on their typical visual strengths, many children will be helped by creating a written checklist or set of pictures that outlines the steps involved in the task. For example, to help a child with taking out the garbage, show pictures of a person removing the garbage bag, tying it, placing it in the can in the garage, and then putting in a new bag. Work through the list with your child several times to help him or her learn the steps involved.

Choosing appropriate tasks is a crucial factor in assigning chores, as we discussed in the last chapter. When first introducing the idea of household responsibilities to your child, start out with a task that is simple and easy to accomplish. Whenever possible, choose tasks that are naturally suited to your child's strengths.

Evan is a 12-year-old boy with high-functioning autism and a preference for order in his physical environment. He has four typically developing siblings, and his home often looks as though a tropical storm has just passed through. His mother decided to assign him the task of organizing the furniture and coffee table in the living room once a day. Evan initially resisted taking on this responsibility, but he reluctantly agreed when he realized it could earn him additional computer time. It soon became clear to his mother that restoring order to the living room actually had a calming effect on Evan. The arrangement enabled him to help out around the house, soothe himself, and earn privileges.

For older children, parents may wish to assign chores that provide practice for skills applicable in a job, such as filing, washing dishes, and preparing the ingredients for cooking.

Homework

Make a structured homework schedule so that your child completes homework at the same time and in the same place every day. Actually putting this information on a visual schedule is helpful. It reminds the child it is coming and also helps the child remember that something more fun will happen after homework is complete. For some children, it may be necessary to further structure the homework session. When a child receives a number of different assignments, he or she may find it challenging to determine the best way to approach the tasks. If your child finds the prospect confusing, help out by making a list of what needs to be done with what priorities. By laying out a concrete plan of attack, you can make the task seem much less overwhelming to children. Chapter 7 contains more detailed suggestions for organizing academic tasks, including homework, for your child.

Many children with AS-HFA are easily distracted. Therefore, they need a workplace that is free from distractions, including noise, clutter, and other family members. Tailor an approach that is appropriate to the attentional capacities and working style of your child. For some children, it is best to complete all homework in a single sitting. Other children find this excessively taxing and may benefit from breaks in between smaller work periods. One parent we worked with sets a kitchen timer for her child. For 30 minutes of productive homework, the child earns a 5-minute computer break. Or you might give your child a break after each assignment or subject is finished. Providing a break or other type of positive reinforcement (maybe a special food treat or a token that can be redeemed for bigger rewards), during or upon completion of homework, will increase your child's motivation. Parents can also make use of the reinforcing properties of homework itself. Many children with AS-HFA are extremely enthusiastic about particular school subjects. Completing favorite homework last serves as reinforcement for working on less interesting subject matter.

Be conscious of the influence that your child's motor and sensory characteristics may have on the homework process. For many children with AS-HFA, handwriting is a difficult fine motor task. The physical difficulty of writing out homework can make the task even more unpleasant. Try to be as creative and flexible as possible in solving these types of problems. For example, ask your child's teacher if he or she could complete the assignment on a computer or dictate the answers rather than write them out (more on these topics in Chapter 7). Children's sensory sensitivities also influence the completion of homework. For some individuals with AS-HFA, reading under certain lighting conditions can be difficult. Experiment with light levels and see what is most comfortable for your child.

Since homework bridges the gap between home and school, the idea of consistency between settings is particularly important. By communicating with your child's teacher, you can learn about strategies that have been successful at school and share techniques that have worked in the home. Communication between parents and teachers also fosters consistency in terms of the rules associated with homework completion. If your child's teacher permits breaks every 20 minutes, then you should use the same schedule at home, rather than a 30-minute break interval. If the teacher reinforces correct work with stickers or check marks, rather than tokens, use those instead. As we mentioned earlier in this chapter, when a child has a single set of rules to follow across multiple settings, he or she has a much easier time knowing what is expected and is more likely to behave accordingly.

Having someone else assist your child with homework, perhaps an academic tutor you hire or a teacher in school, can be very helpful. Some children with Asperger syndrome or high-functioning autism work so slowly that they bring home a great deal of homework. You may find it helpful to request an extra study hall or extra time in the resource room to help your child get more homework done at school. A designated person to help your child structure an approach to homework and to help with the actual completion of homework assignments can be a valuable support. This eliminates one potential area of difficulty that parents must negotiate with their child and also provides parents with some "down time" of their own after a long workday, be it in an office or in the home. Many tutors with experience in working with children with autism spectrum disorders are available, and they can help devise novel strategies for working with your child. Your local autism society probably maintains a list of tutors. Or check with the pediatrics or child psychiatry department of your local hospital or the agency at which your child was diagnosed.

Maintaining a Healthy Family Attitude

Siblings

Working to ensure the psychological well-being of the siblings of children with autism spectrum disorders is one of the most valuable investments parents can make. With a healthy attitude, siblings can be a parent's greatest allies in caring for a child with AS-HFA. They can also be great friends to and serve as role models for children with AS-HFA, particularly for helping them to understand the social world. Finally, of course, when they are happy and feel supported, siblings contribute to the overall well-being of the whole family.

For some typically developing children who have siblings with special needs, there doesn't seem to be much cause for concern. One young lady recently quoted in a national newsletter remarked that just because her brother had special needs, it didn't mean that she did. Her unwavering love for her autistic brother and her candor with peers rendered it an insignificant issue for her. Unfortunately, for many children a sibling with special needs presents a host of familial, social, and personal challenges.

Communicating with Siblings

The most important principles in dealing with siblings of children with AS-HFA are honesty, education, and open-mindedness. Your typically developing child will likely have myriad questions about his or her sibling. Why doesn't he talk to me? Why does she do those weird things? How come he won't play with me? Does she hate me? Can I "catch" autism? Does my brother have Asperger syndrome because I wrestled too hard with him when he was a baby? The more your typical child understands about autism spectrum disorders, the greater the insight into his or her sibling and the less likely that misconceptions, such as those regarding contagion or causality, can contribute to stress. Make sure to create time for open, honest, nonjudgmental discussions when your child can discuss feelings, both positive and negative, regarding his or her sibling with AS-HFA. In these conversations, probe your child regarding his or her experiences at home and at school. What are the issues he or she doesn't understand? What positive and negative aspects of having a brother or sister with AS-HFA has he or she experienced recently? As a parent, you can set an excellent example, being positive and accepting of your child's special needs, but also making clear that sometimes frustration or other negative emotion is unavoidable. A recent study showed that even after parents had talked with their typically developing children about autism spectrum disorders, most of the siblings harbored many misconceptions or didn't understand some basics of the condition. In other words, just because you explain something to your typically developing child, it doesn't mean that he or she has comprehended what you have said. Asking your typically developing child to explain in his or her own words what you have said may be helpful. And having frequent, ongoing discussions, rather than only a few brief conversations, is needed.

A positive approach to facilitating communication with your typically developing child is to include him or her in discussions of how best to help your child with AS-HFA. This is not appropriate for children at all developmental levels, but mature children and adolescents can contribute excellent insights to the experiences of their sibling with AS-HFA and the causes of certain behaviors. As a peer, the sibling may also have helpful opinions about social relationship strategies and school settings. By including your typically developing child in the process, you foster family unity and prevent anyone from feeling excluded.

Guilt and Excessive Responsibility

Some siblings of children with special needs can be excessively demanding of themselves. They might try to help out to the extent that their own schoolwork or social life suffers. Some psychologists speak of the "little parent" effect, in which a typical sibling starts behaving more like a care-giving adult than a child. You can help prevent this by being careful not to rely too much on your typical child's assistance in caring for the sibling with AS-HFA at home or at school.

Typical siblings can also become emotionally vulnerable because of their own thought processes. A certain degree of tension between siblings is natural, even adaptive, in that it provides a forum for learning to resolve conflicts with others. However, a well-intentioned sibling of a child with special needs may experience guilt regarding negative feelings toward a sibling who "just can't help it." Try to help your child understand that these feelings are natural and that what is most important is how he or she acts on them. It is okay, even normal, to resent a brother or sister who requires much of Mom and Dad's attention or who seems to have much lower demands made on him or her. Let your typically developing children know that you understand these thoughts, perhaps even share them sometimes, and that you love them just the same as if all their thoughts of their sibling were warm and positive. Be clear that it is okay to have these thoughts as long as they are not acted on in a harmful or negative way.

Equal Attention, Activity, and Discipline

A common perception of typically developing siblings is that brothers and sisters with autism or Asperger syndrome receive disproportionate amounts of parental attention. Very often, this may be the case. There is no getting around the fact that children with AS-HFA have special needs and may require additional attention to accomplish things typically developing children can do easily. Nevertheless, there are several strategies you can use to prevent siblings' feelings of neglect and potential resentment. In two-parent homes, divide and conquer, splitting up so that you can attend to two children simultaneously. In one-parent families, calling on the assistance of friends or relatives to help out can provide additional caregivers and allow you more flexibility in distributing your time. It is important to be honest and straightforward and to acknowledge your devotion to your typically developing child and your commitment to making sure that all the wheels, not just the squeaky ones, get some grease. Take some time each day to devote your full attention to your typically developing children, even if only briefly. During bedtime routines or other evening activities, make sure that you ask your typically developing children about their experiences, feelings, and concerns. Designate a day once or twice a month that will be devoted to your typical child's interests and find someone else to take care of your child with high-functioning autism or Asperger syndrome on those days. This type of gesture goes a long way in making clear that all your children are important to you.

This last strategy relates to another common sentiment among siblings of children with AS-HFA, the notion that the child's special needs will restrict the activities of the entire family. Take the example of a family outing to a combination pizzeria/arcade. For many children this is about as fun as it gets, but for some children with AS-HFA the noise, visual stimulation, and crowds of people can be overwhelming. It is easy for a parent to avoid such activities to suit the needs of the family member with AS-HFA. However, this practice can foster resentment in typical children. It also reduces the range of experiences encountered by your child with AS-HFA and may reinforce his or her behavioral inflexibility. For this reason, it is essential that you plan a variety of activities that encompass everyone's interests. Allowing the preferences of your child with AS-HFA to dictate family experiences is a dangerous but easy routine to fall into.

Discipline is another area in which it can be difficult to be fair to all of your children. It is sometimes necessary to have different rules and expectations for your child with AS-HFA. This can quite easily foster the impression in typical siblings that a brother or sister with special needs is allowed to misbehave with seeming impunity. There are two strategies for confronting this problem. The first is to critically evaluate your application of disciplinary rules. Maybe your child is right and you are making it a bit easier on your child with AS-HFA. Examine house rules to make sure any discrepancies in expectation across siblings are genuinely necessary. For example, if your typical child has to do chores to earn privileges, make sure your affected child has household responsibilities too, even if they are more basic. Second, when differences exist with justifiable reason, explain the situation to your typical child. A child who understands the reasons for disparities is less likely to resent parents and affected siblings.

Peer Relationships

Many parents express concern regarding the effects that a child with AS-HFA might have on siblings' peer relationships. We've found that peers' responses can range from cruel to caring. Teaching your typical child to explain AS-HFA to others and to express his or her feelings about the subject provides tools for interacting with others on this topic in more comfortable ways. Although it will be important to consult with your typical child before doing so, it can help to invite over some friends from school to meet the affected sibling. This serves to quench their curiosity and help them gain a more realistic perception of autism spectrum disorders. Once classmates understand what their friend's brother or sister is like, they are more likely to act as allies if others are behaving inappropriately and will be more accessible and informed sources of support for your typically developing child. They will also grow up to be more caring, compassionate adults who tolerate diversity.

Some parents find it necessary to set boundaries regarding interaction between an affected sibling and a typical sibling's friends. There's a delicate balance between giving the child with AS-HFA the benefit of social exposure and allowing your typical child to feel independent in his or her friendships. Create certain times when all the children can interact together, for example, by serving a snack or by allowing them to play video games or sports in a group. Also ensure that your typical child has the opportunity to be alone with his or her friends. Some parents find it helpful to make a rule that when children are in common space it is common time, but when friends go into a child's room, it becomes personal time. Respecting your typical child's friendships is important to promote both healthy social development and maintenance of a positive attitude toward the family and affected siblings.

Personal Life

We've already discussed strategies for accommodating household routines to your child with AS-HFA. The same policy is important for your typically developing child. Try to be aware of how your child with AS-HFA affects the household experience of your other children. Is the affected child making too much noise when siblings are trying to sleep or do homework? Make sure you respect the habits and needs of all members of the family.

We've heard numerous children complain about their sibling with AS-HFA taking their belongings and failing to respect their personal space. Given the difficulties children with AS-HFA experience in judging personal boundaries and inferring the sentiments of others, it is important for you to intervene and make sure that your typical child has a "safe" space where prized possessions or personal items can be kept away from prying eyes and probing hands. This space can be a drawer, a closet, or even a room that is off limits to his or her sibling. In addition to the practical advantage of providing your child with a safe spot, it sends a clear message that you are keeping your typical child's interests in mind. When implementing this idea, be consistent and provide your AS-HFA child with a special and safe space for his or her treasures too!

Additional Support

There are several books that focus specifically on sibling issues. *Siblings of Children with Autism*, by Sandra L. Harris, PhD, provides specific strategies for teaching children about autism and helping them communicate their experiences on the subject. A number of age-appropriate books and websites are designed to help siblings of children with autism spectrum disorders grapple with the unique challenges the situation presents (see the Appendix). Sometimes counseling is a helpful source of support for the typically developing child experiencing difficulty coming to terms with his or her sibling's disability. Some care settings provide support groups specifically designed for siblings of children with autism or Asperger syndrome. These groups provide a comfortable, friendly setting for children to learn from and make friends with others who have had similar experiences.

Parents as People

Autism spectrum disorders are recognized as some of the most difficult diagnoses for parents to come to terms with. Perhaps because we know so little about their cause, many parents instinctively feel a sense of guilt. Depression in parents after receiving the diagnosis is not uncommon. Marital relationships are strained, resulting in higher than average rates of divorce among families of children with special needs. Thus, it is important that you consider not only the needs of your children but also your own needs. You are the primary support for your child with AS-HFA, and the healthier you are, the better support you will be able to provide.

One ingredient in taking care of yourself is to invest some time, even if it is just a few minutes after everyone is asleep, in personal activities every day. Preserve your individual identity beyond being the parent of a child with special needs. Take turns with your spouse taking a night off once a week to pursue personal recreation or socialize with friends. If you are a single parent, try to arrange for a babysitter or friend to care for your children once a week so you can take a break for personal socializing or other individual pursuits.

Just as an individual's mental health can suffer if it is neglected, a relationship requires similar attention. It can be very difficult for parents to preserve quality time with a partner. Continually neglecting the relationship can have adverse effects on everyone in the family, including the child you are working so hard to help. Many parents call on relatives or friends to watch the children for a few hours each week. Other parents hire respite providers to allow them a few hours of personal or social time. An essential means of minimizing stress in two-parent families is to thoroughly discuss and agree on treatment and parenting decisions, both to minimize discord and to achieve consistency. Sometimes this is difficult and you may find it necessary to involve a professional, such as your child's doctor, to discuss different options and treatment decisions.

Maintaining adult relationships can be even more difficult when one of the partners is not the biological parent of the child with AS-HFA. Single parents who are dating or in new relationships often feel torn about taking time away from their child. We can't stress enough that taking care of yourself rivals taking care of your child in importance. If you are lonely, unfulfilled, and in dire need of adult conversation, your patience and resources for your AS-HFA child will diminish. Try hard to carve out special time, away from your child, to interact with other adults, including romantic partners. You may find it helpful to provide information about AS-HFA to new partners in small doses, if they appear interested. Encourage interactions with your child with AS-HFA in structured circumstances that highlight his or her skills. The stereotypes of severe autism that many people hold, just because they know no better, are important to dispel for anyone who may become important in your life. Help others learn about the unique and interesting side of AS-HFA. As you know, living with AS-HFA is not always easy, but it is by no means always difficult either.

Whether yours is a one-parent or a two-parent family, you should take advantage of the numerous support groups that have been formed for parents of children with autism spectrum disorders. These groups can usually offer useful tips from parents who have encountered comparable challenges. Some groups also provide child care while parents meet, which gives parents some much needed "down time" and creates an informal social group for children with AS-HFA. The most important benefit of support groups, however, is the opportunity to communicate with others who have survived the same struggles you are encountering. It can be very reassuring to realize your situation is not as extraordinary as it may often seem and to learn successful coping strategies from empathic peers.

If you can't find a support group in your area, consider creating an informal group. Several parents who have participated in social skills groups at the University of Washington have gone on to form informal support/social skills groups on their own. Meeting at a family's home once a month gives parents a chance to discuss issues and provide support for one another. This group also hires an experienced graduate student to watch the children while they meet, so that the children receive some social skills guidance during their interactions.

Managing a family with a child with AS-HFA puts extra stress on everyone, to be sure. However, by using the strategies in this chapter, we hope that your family can more easily focus on the opportunities for accomplishment, joy, and laughter that your special child can inspire as well.

CHAPTER 7

Asperger Syndrome and High-Functioning Autism at School

At age 8, Joseph is the best reader and speller in his third-grade class—so far ahead of his classmates, in fact, that he joins the sixth graders for English. He is also a whiz at computers and often is able to figure out the problem when his teacher has trouble logging on or opening folders. His teacher, who is very fond of Joseph and continually amazed at his talents, asks him to help a classmate who has had little experience with computers. Joseph beams as he demonstrates how to use the mouse to point and click. In a recent talent show, Joseph showed his class how he can read the *New York Times* upside down in a mirror. Joseph struggles in many other areas, however. He sometimes misinterprets what he reads and often can't answer simple questions about a paragraph that he has read aloud quickly and flawlessly. Joseph can subtract three-digit numbers in his head but can't figure out how much money he needs for lunch or if he gets the right amount of change back. His handwriting is very poor and he resists using a pencil, so his teacher allows him to use a keyboard for writing assignments. His desk is a horrible mess, with papers that he has forgotten to hand in, assignments he has never finished, old food, and little trinkets spilling out. He often appears as if he isn't listening or is absorbed in daydreams. When the teacher gives directions, Joseph sits quietly, lost in thought, while all around him his classmates get their workbooks out and turn to the page the teacher indicated. And Joseph often complains of boredom when the class studies topics that don't interest him (basically anything unrelated to geography). His parents have asked the teacher to modify some of his assignments so that they somehow involve geography, but the teacher is not sure whether this will go too far in "coddling" Joseph or making him stand out even further from his classmates.

When Hans Asperger first described children like Joseph, he highlighted both their special cognitive strengths and their serious academic weaknesses, saying that "these exceptional human beings must be given exceptional educational treatment. . . . These children raise questions of central importance to psychology and education." He recognized immediately that standard educational practices would not always work for children with Asperger syndrome (and high-functioning autism) and that special measures would need to be taken to ensure that they achieved to their true potential. He believed that if this was done, children with these conditions were capable of "a high level of original thought and experience" and "exceptional achievements in later life." In this chapter, we outline a variety of different school services and accommodations that use the special strengths of the condition to help children and adolescents with autism spectrum disorders succeed academically, despite the cognitive challenges of these conditions.

The Cognitive and Academic Profile of Individuals with AS-HFA

Chapter 5 reviewed the cognitive talents that are often part of high-functioning autism and Asperger syndrome, and Chapter 2 introduced the cognitive challenges that are part of the diagnostic profile for autism spectrum disorders. Joseph exemplifies a typical (although not universal) pattern, in which some of his academic skills are highly advanced, others are age-appropriate, and still others are truly deficient. Joseph can sound out almost any word he is shown, but he doesn't always know what it means. This indicates a dissociation between his reading decoding and reading comprehension skills. Similarly, in math he understands the rules of addition and subtraction and is even beginning to memorize the multiplication tables, but he has trouble applying these skills to the real world and using them in a commonsense fashion. He often appears unmotivated to learn about things that other children are intrinsically interested in. Earning good grades and obtaining teacher and parent approval seem unimportant to Joseph.

One of Joseph's greatest sources of difficulty is his trouble with organization, planning, and goal-directed activities (often called "executive function" skills). Joseph frequently daydreams, which causes him to miss what the teacher is saying or what he is supposed to be doing. He is not distracted by external stimuli, however, as in the case of individuals with attention-deficit/hyperactivity disorder (ADHD), but internally: he can get totally absorbed in his own thoughts and lose track of what is going on in the classroom. Joseph also has trouble managing time and works very slowly and methodically; consequently, he often falls behind during class, resulting in hours of homework in the evening. He can't seem to get organized: when he sits down to do homework, he has invariably forgotten something he needs to complete the assignment. Either he's left it at school or he goes off in search of it and gets distracted by something of higher interest and an hour elapses. Joseph's backpack is such a jumble that he can't find the homework he's done to turn it in—or else he just plain forgets that this last step is essential. In mid-February, he gave his family a Christmas ornament he had made in school as a holiday gift after discovering it at the bottom of his desk. Joseph tends to get bogged down in details and has trouble distinguishing what is most relevant from minor issues. He is prone to go off on tangents or to get overly focused on something unimportant. For example, when writing a book report, he spent so much time trying to figure out the author's date of birth that he wasn't able to complete the assignment, even though his mother stayed up until midnight to help him with it.

This profile of strengths and weaknesses is quite distinct from the learning disabilities that teachers are most often aware of. For example, children with dyslexia (reading disability), the most common learning disorder, demonstrate essentially the opposite pattern from Joseph. They are unable to sound out words due to a profound deficit in hearing speech sounds in language and difficulty learning how letters correspond to sounds. When asked to read aloud, they read haltingly and with great difficulty, mispronouncing, skipping, or guessing at many words. Despite these problems, children with dyslexia can answer questions about what they've read perfectly—an absolutely uncanny ability considering all the reading errors they have made and the basic lack of correspondence between the printed page and what they say aloud.

This is the kind of pattern that teachers learn about during their training and know how to treat. But many teachers have never been faced with a student who can read a passage perfectly but has trouble understanding what it means. Likewise, organizational and planning difficulties are not typical forms of learning disability. Teachers often have trouble believing that a child who is bright in so many ways can "forget" about a long-planned field trip or fail to anticipate what materials are needed to complete an assignment. Because of the relative rarity of these academic difficulties, children with AS-HFA can frustrate even the most understanding teachers and parents. Occasionally this leads to misinterpretation of the child's behaviors and negative attributions about the student—for example, that he or she is lazy, stubborn, willfully disobedient or defiant. Many teachers, and even some parents, have felt that the child "could do it if he [she] really wanted to." This can be a harmful attitude for the child. It not only can set up an adversarial relationship between the child and the teacher, but, even worse, may prevent the child from getting the services or accommodations he or she might need to succeed in school and later in life. Finally, this attitude can also have a negative effect on your child's self-esteem and feelings about school.

Learning Disabilities and AS-HFA

The fact that there are major distinctions between the cognitive challenges posed by autism spectrum disorders and those posed by learning disabilities does not preclude the possibility that a child will have both. While it is relatively uncommon for children with autism spectrum disorders to have dyslexia too, it does occasionally happen. If your child is experiencing trouble with phonics, by all means have him or her evaluated for dyslexia. Most school psychologists and many clinical psychologists in the community are trained to perform these specialized evaluations.

One learning disability is actually somewhat common among children with autism spectrum disorders. It is known as nonverbal learning disability, or NLD. As discussed in Chapter 2, children with NLD experience selective difficulty with mathematics, visual–spatial skills (for example, completing puzzles, mazes, drawing), and handwriting, but function fine when the activity relies primarily on language skills (for example, reading, spelling, answering questions). They are often clumsy and late to walk or develop other motor skills, such as riding a bike. Many children with NLD have trouble reading the emotions of others and may have other social difficulties, such as shyness or trouble making friends. Some of these difficulties overlap with the autism spectrum disorders (social problems and delayed motor skills, for example), while others are relatively rare in autism spectrum disorders (such as poor visual–spatial skills). To be diagnosed with NLD, a child must experience the hallmark cognitive and academic symptoms of the syndrome, including poor math and visual–spatial skills and lowered nonverbal intelligence; the social and motor symptoms alone are not enough for a diagnosis. Dr. Ami Klin and Dr. Fred Volkmar, researchers at Yale University, have found that the NLD pattern is more common in children with Asperger syndrome than in those with high-functioning autism, although it is clearly not universal in Asperger syndrome and *is* occasionally seen in high-functioning autism. If your child exhibits several of these difficulties, it is worth requesting an evaluation from your school to see if he or she would benefit from extra assistance in learning math or qualify for occupational therapy services.

Educational Placement

One of the first questions raised by parents of children who have been diagnosed with Asperger syndrome or high-functioning autism involves school placement. Would their child be better off in a regular or in a special education classroom? Are classrooms for children with autism spectrum disorders better than those for children with more general learning or behavior problems? Should they investigate private schools? The answers to these questions depend on the individual child: there is no placement that is universally successful for all children with AS-HFA. The rule of thumb is that a child who is performing at or close to grade level and displays relatively few challenging behaviors (for example, outbursts, aggression, interrupting) can benefit from education in a regular classroom. However, even when these conditions are met, there is some risk that these children will fall between the cracks. Regular classrooms have a much higher student-to-teacher ratio than special education settings. When the child doesn't understand something, he or she will be unlikely to seek help or clarification, and teachers may be too busy with the larger group to notice. His or her problems in comprehension, abstract reasoning, and organization may go unrecognized if the child has good reading and calculation skills. Teasing may not be monitored, and development of social skills may not be a focus of remediation as it might be in a special education classroom. So even children who seem to have natural AS-HFA strengths to benefit from and relatively minimal challenges to impede regular education will likely still need some special accommodations to help them be successful.

To reiterate a theme from Chapter 4, *your active participation in your child's educational program is essential*. You are an expert on your child. You understand his or her strengths, interests, routines, triggers, and what has and has not worked for him or her in the past. School personnel, on the other hand, are specialists in academic policies, classroom settings and options, educational principles, and grade-appropriate curricula. The old adage "two heads are better than one" is particularly apt in this situation, so actively collaborate with your child's teachers and principal in setting up educational goals and a curriculum. Your job is a tough one, because you must walk a fine line between advocating for your child's special needs (which may be more obvious to you than to his or her teachers and the school administrators) and working *with* the school in a collegial and professional fashion. Choose your battles and be willing to compromise. This is easier said than done, we know, but it is very important to try to prevent the development of an adversarial relationship with your child's school since, in our experience, this *never* helps your child.

Special Education Options—and What Is an IEP?

Since the 1970s, federal legislation has required states to provide equal educational opportunities to all children with disabilities. In 1975, the U.S. Congress passed Public Law 94-142, which established the basic right to a "free and appropriate public education" for children with disabilities. In addition, this congressional bill mandated that schools provide a fair and unbiased evaluation to determine eligibility for services and place children in the "least restrictive" setting that could meet

Steps in Finding the Right Program
for Your Child

1. As soon as you receive the diagnosis, contact the principal of your child's school.

   - Explain the test results.
   - Ask for a referral to the school personnel who conduct eligibility determinations for special education.

2. After determining if your child is eligible for special education, find out about different classroom options in your district.

   - Visit the different classrooms and interview the teachers.
   - Ask about the availability of certain accommodations or the willingness to provide them.

3. If your child is not eligible for special education, request an appointment with the district's "504 Coordinator."

   - Request a 504 evaluation.
   - Ask about the availability of certain accommodations or the willingness to provide them.

4. If finances permit it, simultaneously investigate private school options.

   - Call your state autism society or the doctor who diagnosed your child for the names of private schools that have worked successfully with AS-HFA children.
   - Visit the different classrooms and interview the teachers.
   - Ask about the availability of certain accommodations or the willingness to provide them.

their educational needs. Specific special education services and goals for the child were to be listed formally in an Individualized Education Program, or IEP. Parents were strongly encouraged to participate in decision making about their child's education by being part of the team that set up the IEP. Although this legislation is almost 30 years old and has undergone a number of amendments (and new names), its spirit remains strong and continues to regulate special education eligibility and delivery of services today. The current law that governs special education, the Individuals with Disabilities Education Act (or IDEA), was reauthorized by the U.S. Senate in 1997.

While these statutes grant specific educational rights to your child, it is important to understand that obtaining these rights involves a very intense process. Many stages and layers of development must be passed through on the way to putting a program into place for an individual child. Through these stages and layers, you may find that your local school is cooperative and open to new ideas, or you may find that the school has a preset agenda and is not willing to compromise. If you reach the latter point, you should be prepared to advocate for your child. It is paramount that you know your rights and responsibilities. Contact your state education department to get information about the special education process in your state.

In the meantime, also be aware that an autism spectrum diagnosis (or indeed *any* psychological or psychiatric diagnosis) does *not* guarantee that your child will qualify for special education services. Eligibility is determined by examining the impact of the condition on your child's academic skills and other areas of functioning in the school setting. Different states implement the federal guidelines in different manners. Most states require a discrepancy between a child's IQ and his or her academic or other functional skills to qualify for special education, but the specific manner in which this discrepancy is calculated and the amount of discrepancy required vary from state to state. After obtaining a diagnosis, parents should bring the diagnostic report (or ask that it be sent) to their child's school and request an evaluation to assess his or her educational needs. It is possible that the results of this evaluation will indicate that your child does not qualify for special education services. If so, don't lose heart—there are other options for receiving support in the school, which are discussed in a later section on classroom accommodations and 504 Plans.

If your child does in fact prove eligible for special education, then an IEP will be prepared, with much input from you. The IEP is best thought of as a contract between parents and schools that outlines what the team agrees is an appropriate education for the child, how it will be delivered, and how it will be evaluated to see if it is working. The IDEA law mandates that a "team" develop, review, and revise the IEP. The IEP team consists of:

1. A school representative (other than teachers) qualified to offer or supervise special education services (if your district has an autism specialist, he or she may serve in this role; alternate possibilities include the director of special education or another school administrator).
2. The child's regular and special education teachers.
3. Other school personnel providing services to the child (for example, occupational and/or speech therapists).
4. Parents.
5. The child, when possible and if age-appropriate.

As a member of the IEP team, you have some choices and some power in the decision-making process, at least more so than you may be accustomed to with your non-special-needs children. If there is something you think your child needs at school (such as language services, social skills training, help with goal setting and organization, reading comprehension tutoring, an aide), your best recourse is to get it put in the IEP. Keep in mind, too, that you can ask to include on the team anyone with special knowledge or expertise concerning the needs of your child.

Know your legal rights. For example, you do not need to sign the IEP until you agree that it provides what the law promises you is important. Equally important, however, is understanding that the law says your child is entitled to an *appropriate* education, not the *best* education. Just as with regular education, parents may choose to "purchase" what they perceive to be the *best* education for their child through a private school. That said, keep in mind that the educational plan must be individualized, that is, specifically tailored to meet the unique needs of your child. This means that the school must develop a unique plan for each student, regardless of what the school offers other children.

What happens if you disagree with your school over the appropriate/best distinction? For example, sometimes parents think that a particular service is *appropriate* for their child with AS-HFA, and therefore should be funded by the school system, but school personnel see this service as *the best* technique, and therefore not something the school is willing to provide. In our experience, a combination of persistence and willingness to negotiate will often get parents fairly close to what they desire in the IEP. If, however, after a series of negotiations with the school, you still feel the program being offered by the school is not appropriate, you can contact your state education department to find out what alternatives are available. The federal government has mandated that every state must have an agency designated to help parents get through the special education process.

IEPs contain specific goals and objectives for your child's education. A *goal* is a general desired change in your child's learning, skills, or behaviors, while an *objective* is the specific definition of that change and how it will be measured. Goals are usually broader and longer term (perhaps set annually), while objectives are shorter term benchmarks for determining if appropriate progress toward the goal is being made. For example, an IEP goal might be "to increase reading comprehension," while a corresponding objective would be "to answer questions about a paragraph accurately 75% of the time." It is important to choose IEP goals and objectives that are both meaningful and realistic. You want the skills specified to be ones that are important to your child's functionality, independence, and later success, while also being attainable. If IEP objectives are set too high, it will appear that your child is "failing" when in fact he or she is really straining to meet an inappropriate skill level. If the objective is set too low, your child may not be receiving the level of assistance and intervention that he or she truly needs. And remember that an IEP is not immutable: at any time, any member of the IEP team (including you as parents) can ask that the IEP be reviewed and revised. This is typically done at least annually and more often if necessary. If objectives are being met at an unanticipated pace or not met at all or if new diagnostic or evaluation results are obtained, then a meeting of the IEP team is warranted.

In addition to specific goals and objectives, IEPs contain a list of related services that will be provided to your child in the school setting, such as speech–language therapy, occupational therapy, adaptive physical education, or social skills training. Some children with AS-HFA need one-on-one instruction for certain academic tasks or during certain activities (for example, groups) when their behavior or understanding may limit their ability to benefit otherwise from the instruction. In such cases, a request for an aide can be made in the IEP. An aide can be full- or part-time and can be assigned to an individual student or shared among a few students who would all benefit from smaller group learning. Aides can be extremely valuable, but they are usually paraprofessionals without any advanced degrees (or perhaps even formal training). Therefore, it is important to request that your aide either have prior experience or receive specific training in both standard educational principles and best practices for students with AS-HFA. It is also important to ensure that your child's aide gives him or her chances to "practice" the skills without always jumping in to help. Too much one-to-one assistance can be as bad as too little. Specifically, it may make your child overly dependent on prompts from an adult and therefore may reduce the child's initiative and ability to function independently. Aides need to know how to provide subtle structure without eliminating chances for the child to interact, practice, and try, before offering more help.

Classroom Options

Children can receive special education services in a self-contained classroom—one whose members all have difficulties of some type and who are all receiving special education—or in regular classrooms, partially or even primarily. In regular classrooms, their IEP goals are implemented by a regular education teacher in collaboration with special education staff. This so-called mainstreaming has the benefit of surrounding the child with typically developing peers and exposing the child to appropriate behavior and good models of age-typical communication and interpersonal relationships. In fact, one basic principle within special education legislation is that children with disabilities should be educated in the "least restrictive environment" (this principle is often nicknamed "LRE" by school staff), alongside children who are not disabled, and that putting children in special classes or removing them from the regular education environment should be minimized. On the other hand, your child may not receive the level of attention he or she needs if he or she spends all his or her school hours in a regular classroom (also called "full inclusion"). Resources, funding, and specialized teacher training are usually greater in special education classes. Thus, you will need to weigh the costs and benefits of some "pull-out" classes or other forms of "segregated" special education for your child. There are no inherent flaws in either setting, but an effort should be made to provide a balance between "normality" and resources for your child's special needs.

There are a variety of different classroom options for children who are educated part or most of the school day in self-contained classrooms. The labels for these classrooms vary from state to state, but most include the following options: classes for children with communication disorders, learning disabilities, behavioral or emotional problems, intellectual deficits, and occasionally autism (although usually these autism units serve more severely affected children with few or no verbal skills). Any of these placements might provide a good option for your child. It will depend on class composition and the functioning level of the other students, the teacher's skill and style, the location of the classroom (within your neighborhood school or not), and other variables. The best way to decide if your child would benefit from some education in one of these self-contained classes is to talk with special education staff about the appropriateness of these classes for your child and then to visit them and talk with the teacher. This is often done in late winter or early spring of the preceding school year, when schools are getting a clearer idea of what the class composition will be and what kinds of space and staffing issues the school may face, as well as some sense of your child's needs and how well he or she fared in the previous year's placement. If your special education staff has not introduced this topic for discussion by March or April, you should ask to set up a meeting to begin transition planning for the next school year.

Public or Private School?

Parents sometimes turn to private schools when they feel that their child's unique needs can't be met by the public school options in their region. Private schools may seem to have a clear advantage since most offer substantially smaller class sizes and more individualized instruction than public schools. But there are other factors to consider. Perhaps the most important is that private schools are not governed by the federal laws that mandate a "free and appropriate" public education. Obviously, private schooling is not free, and private schools are not required to provide "appropriate" services. So keep in mind that a move to a private school will involve relinquishing your legal right to these services. But some private schools will agree to provide certain accommodations, and some even specialize in such accommodations, in which case such a school may well be a good setting for your child.

Another consideration, however, is the uniformity and homogeneity of the school. In some private schools there is so little diversity and the student body is so geared toward high achievement that the child with AS-HFA stands out far more than in a public school. In some private schools, it can be so much harder to fit in that it is not worth the other benefits the setting might offer.

Finally, money is often an issue. Many families need to choose among a variety of therapeutic options and must constantly weigh the costs against the benefits. Will this money be better spent elsewhere? If we choose this private school, will we need to give up speech therapy or social skills training? This is another example of the need to "choose your battles."

Parents sometimes ask where the best schools for children with autism spectrum disorders are located in the country, expressing a willingness to move if their child's needs could be better met elsewhere. The simple answer is that there aren't any—or at least any that advertise themselves as national schools just or primarily for students with AS-HFA. And, as this and other chapters should make clear, it might not be such a good thing to have your child segregated not only in a special class but also in a special school, with no typical peers available to serve as models and potential friends. If you do find a special school of this type in the future, be sure that it provides opportunities for inclusion and education with nondisabled students as well. The principle of the "least restrictive environment" is not just legal policy but is also good for your child's social development.

Classroom Accommodations—and What Is a 504 Plan?

As mentioned above, all is not lost if your child does not qualify for special education and an IEP. The Federal Rehabilitation Act of 1973 is a law that protects the civil and constitutional rights of people with disabilities. Section 504 of this law (since renamed the Americans with Disabilities Act, or ADA) mandates access to a free and appropriate public education for all people with disabilities. Disabilities are broadly defined in this legislation (more broadly than in IDEA, the special education law) as any limit in any major life activity, including "learning."

At first, this law was interpreted as an obligation to provide *physical* access to education for people with disabilities (for example, curb cuts and elevators for students in wheelchairs, sign language interpreters for deaf students, and the like). More recently, however, the meaning of "access" to an appropriate education has been expanded. Section 504 has increasingly been used to secure services for children with disabilities who don't qualify for special education but still have educational needs (or, in the language of the law, "limits in learning"). All school districts have a designated "504 coordinator" who helps put together services for children qualified under Section 504. In brief, a "504 Plan" is a written document that lays out a variety of modifications that a child needs to be successful in a regular education environment. Usually these accommodations are somewhat less time-consuming and require less intensive intervention and fewer trained staff to implement them than those provided via an IEP. The downside to 504 Plans (relative to IEPs) is that there is no federal funding to implement them; thus, whatever you ask your school to provide in a 504 Plan must be done with existing money (usually taken from somewhere else) or at no additional cost. In the following sections, we outline a variety of interventions and accommodations that can be added to a 504 Plan to help your child succeed (not just survive) in school, despite the learning and/or behavioral difficulties imposed by having an autism spectrum disorder. It is also worth mentioning that these very same accommodations can be part of an IEP (in other words, 504 goals are not mutually exclusive of IEP goals) if your child qualifies for special education under IDEA.

Teacher and Classroom Characteristics

One of the most important ingredients in a successful school program is the teacher—specifically, the teacher's level of flexibility, open-mindedness, positive attitude, sense of humor, and willingness to try new things. Teachers who value diversity, accept students as they are, and enjoy the uniqueness of those with AS-HFA are particularly valuable. You may find these qualities in teachers in regular classrooms, self-contained special education classrooms, or private schools. The following characteristics are often seen in the classrooms of teachers who have successfully served children with AS-HFA (and with other special needs):

- Consistent routines and rules.
- Consistent places that assignment materials are kept and assignments are collected.
- A posted classroom schedule.
- Use of clear, simple, unambiguous language.
- Provision of written instructions (such as directions written on the chalkboard).
- Preferential desk placement near the teacher and away from distractions, such as windows or corridors.
- A special work station when noise or other distractions disrupt work.
- Allocation of sufficient time for instructions, repetition of instructions, and individual student assistance.
- Frequent monitoring of student work pace and work product.
- Directing of questions toward the student to see that he or she understands the work and is attending.
- Immediate feedback on performance, including reinforcement for both effort and productivity.

Some school districts will allow parents to visit several classrooms and hand-pick a teacher and classroom that possess these qualities, whether it is in the child's neighborhood school or not. And many teachers who do not already do these things will be willing to, if asked. Many of these things will benefit all students in the class and are not particularly time-consuming for the teacher. They are prime examples of the kinds of modifications that can be listed in your child's 504 Plan (or an IEP).

A wide variety of additional accommodations that may help your child can be added to a 504 Plan (or an IEP). Some of these are, in contrast to the preceding list, more work for a teacher who may already be juggling a large class and be terribly overworked. Some of these accommodations may draw unwanted attention to your child and make him or her stand out in a way that turns out to be unacceptable to you or the teachers. Sometimes school personnel worry that providing a service to one child will open the floodgates to similar requests for other children, and who therefore resist your request for the accommodation. Also remember that there is no extra funding coming to your school to pay for the modifications listed in a 504 Plan. For all these reasons, it is important to choose judiciously from the ideas presented below and ask specifically for those that you feel will truly be helpful for your child.

Workload

You may find that your child has hours of homework each evening, perhaps much more than other students in the class. This may be due to his or her slow work habits and inefficiency that result from being preoccupied by special interests or distracted by details, as well as by the poorly developed concept of time so often seen in children with AS-HFA. This often places a large burden on parents, because your child will likely need a great deal of structure and supervision from you to finish this homework. We saw a couple in our clinic that who were so stressed by their son's hours of homework and his resistance to completing it that it created terrible friction between them and eventually (combined with other stresses) led to their divorce. If your situation is in any way similar, even if not quite so extreme, you may want to ask your child's teacher to consider some of the following options for managing time.

If your child seems unaware of passing time, then an intervention as simple as providing a kitchen timer or watch with an alarm can be used to help your child monitor his or her work pace. These devices provide concrete cues for the beginning and end of each work activity, as well as advance warnings of deadlines. Another option that may be necessary is decreasing your child's workload. Perhaps the number of problems required could be reduced (for example, your child must complete 10 math problems instead of the 20 his or her classmates must finish) or the length of the assignment decreased (writing one versus four paragraphs on a particular topic). If your child can still learn a concept without doing quite so many problems, this may be a possibility. Another option is to have less information on a page so that the amount of work *appears* less, even if it truly is not. A child faced with one page of 10 math problems may be overwhelmed, but the same child who faces a few pages of less dense problems (perhaps three per page) may find the work manageable. When your child reaches junior and senior high school and perhaps college, an additional version of this principle is to limit the number of courses he or she takes. It may be best for him or her to enroll in two to three classes per semester, instead of the usual four or five especially when he or she is taking time-consuming or difficult classes. We also recommend enrolling in small classes, where the amount of attention from the professor may be greater. Or your child may want to choose less popular classes (we know a college student with AS-HFA who chose to take Russian instead of Spanish), where class size may be smaller and professors may be highly motivated to retain students. It is more important for your child to have a successful experience than to follow a typical schedule. You may also want to ask that certain curriculum requirements be waived, especially those that prove difficult for most people with autism spectrum disorders, like advanced math and foreign language classes.

Visual Strategies

As we've highlighted throughout this book, children and adolescents with AS-HFA are often visual learners. Thus, providing as much visual input and structure as possible will help most students with AS-HFA. For example, teachers could be asked to write instructions they give to the whole class on the chalkboard, so that if your child is not paying attention for a moment or cannot process the verbal instructions quickly, he or she has a record and reminder of what to do. The teacher might also provide your child with individual instructions, in the form of a written prompt or reminder on an index card that can be taped to his or her desk. Another example of providing visual structure is to show your child a model of the final goal or completed product. It is often easier to work toward the conclusion when the child can *see* what he or she is supposed to be doing than if the end product is abstract or otherwise intangible.

Executive Function Help

Several strategies can be used to compensate for organization and planning difficulties, also called *executive function problems,* that your child may demonstrate. One is a *weekly homework log* that is sent from school to home and back, keeping all parties informed of work due and progress on it. A description of the homework and the due date are entered in the log by your child, often with the teacher's help. Teachers may need to check that your child has all homework and associated materials before leaving school. Parents can then enter their initials in the log to indicate that their child has worked on the assignment at home, and teachers can sign off when it has been turned in. Teachers can indicate grades received as well as the number of times that homework was not completed on time. You may also want to request that teachers give your child advance warning of upcoming due dates, even before other students in the class, so that he or she has extra time to complete the assignment.

Assignment checklists can be used to help break large, often over-whelming, tasks into manageable units. For example, an assignment checklist might contain information about how to get started ("Begin with question 7 on page 4"), what to do (every other item, for example), how to recognize when the task is complete ("Finish 10 problems"), where to store or hand in the completed product (for example, a back-pack near the door), and a reminder to clean up. For larger assign-ments, timelines might be supplied along with a list of subgoals. For ex-ample, if your child has a book report due at the end of the month, you or the teacher could not only break this large goal into its smaller ob-jectives (visit library, choose book, read book, outline main ideas, and so on), but assign due dates for each of these subgoals. Otherwise, your child may start the process only a day or two in advance since he hasn't realized the length of time that each of the smaller goals will require. It is also helpful to provide a list of materials needed for each assignment (perhaps a calculator, specific assignment sheet, the correct book, a writing implement). While this may seem obvious, one of the most common reasons that students with AS-HFA fail to complete work is that they don't have the appropriate materials ready when they sit down to work.

Day planners, simplified versions of the kind that many adults use, can also help organize your child. All events with a designated time should be entered in the planner, including, for example, time to wake up, eat breakfast, and get to the bus stop; time for major school activi-ties and after-school appointments; and times for dinner, homework, relaxation, and bed. Children enjoy it when an empty box is placed next to each item, to be filled with a check mark or sticker once the activity has been completed. This provides a visual concrete cue identifying completed and upcoming events. Since day planners are relatively widely used and do not make the child stand out from peers, they tend to be well accepted. It may also be helpful for parents to adopt a day planner themselves, modeling its use for their child. Also, including things your child likes or considers special, such as calculators, favorite writing implements, money, or trading cards, in a pouch in the day planner can increase its relevance and worth, reducing the likelihood that it will be "forgotten" at home or school.

"To do" lists can be included in the day planner for tasks that need to get done but do not have specific designated times (errands, telephone calls, chores, and so on). You'll need to teach your child to cross out items as they are completed, and then each evening to transfer items that have yet to be finished to the next day's list. Items on the list can be prioritized with a numbering or color-coding system.

Help-Seeking Routines

Because of their social difficulties and their difficulty initiating interactions, students with AS-HFA often do not ask for help when they need it. Therefore, it is important for teachers to be on the lookout for the need for help, to check in with your child periodically to monitor work, and to create signals or other routines that your child can use to indicate the need for help. Sometimes this can be as simple as teaching the child to raise his hand. If a child is particularly self-conscious and unlikely to call attention to himself in this way, however, the teacher could supply a specific but unobtrusive behavior that the child could use to signal the need for help—perhaps turning sideways, with feet toward the aisle rather than directly under the desk, or placing a special object on the desktop.

Group Learning

Social difficulties can also present an obstacle to group work for the child with AS-HFA. Since the 1990s, the educational principle of collaborative learning has been prominent in American schools. Children work in groups to complete a common product. The goal of this type of instruction is learning to work together, to negotiate, and to help one another. It is not sufficient for each child to focus on his or her individual goal or part of the task; one weak link, and the whole project will receive a lower grade. This practice appears to have many obvious educational and less tangible social benefits. However, as you might imagine, this kind of work is very hard for the average child with AS-HFA. At the worst, it can mean that your child does not learn particular concepts because the learning process so much depends on social skills. If so, you may find it necessary to request another learning format (such as individual assignments) for your child. On the other hand, if your child shows some ability to participate in group exercises, they can be great social opportunities.

Difficulties can also arise when students are expected to work in self-chosen pairs or teams. It can be exceedingly painful to be the only one "not picked," a not uncommon situation for students with AS-HFA. In such circumstances, parents can encourage teachers to draw numbers or use some other means of pairing off in classes.

Handwriting Alternatives

Many people with autism spectrum disorders have poor handwriting. It can be very difficult to read, as well as slow and laborious to produce. As Clint, the young adult with high-functioning autism you met in Part I of this book, lamented, "It's like having a Pentium III processor hooked up to a dot matrix printer." This often results in anxiety, resistance to activities that must be handwritten, and even some of the challenging behaviors we described in the last chapter. To alleviate some of these problems, you can ask that your child's teacher provide extra time for and/or shorten written assignments. Also, it's important that your child be graded on content, not the neatness or legibility of his or her script. You can also ask your child's teacher to allow him or her to submit work in an alternative form (typed on a computer, audiotaped, dictated to a peer or parent), with the exception of those tasks that were designed specifically to promote and develop handwriting. Many schools now provide access to laptop computers or to keyboards that are connected to a central classroom computer and printer.

Labored handwriting makes note taking difficult for students with AS-HFA (as does their slower auditory processing and their tendency to become preoccupied with details and special interests). It is very helpful if teachers give a copy of their notes or an outline of the class discussion to students with AS-HFA (preferably beforehand), so that they can listen to lectures and concentrate on what the teacher adds while speaking, without the frustration of taking notes. Another possibility is asking that a peer provide copies of his or her notes to the child or teen with AS-HFA. Permitting tape-recording of lectures is another method to assist with note taking. Similarly, copying from the chalkboard can be a challenge (due not only to writing problems but also to the child's need to constantly switch back and forth between two tasks:

reading and writing). Access to teacher or classmate notes will significantly reduce this problem too. Some parents worry that these accommodations will place an unnecessary spotlight on their child. In our experience, however, these academic modifications can make your child fit in better, and in the long run actually reduce the spotlight on your child. At the college level, it is the rule rather than the exception that teachers provide lecture outlines to students, so you might encourage your child's teachers to provide the notes to everyone in the class, not just the student with high-functioning autism or Asperger syndrome.

Test Taking

Tests are another academic activity that often present special challenges to the child with AS-HFA, due to the combination of time management, handwriting, anxiety, and executive function problems. The student could be permitted to take exams in an alternative format (for example, orally, or by using a fill-in-the-blanks written format), to have extra time for tests, and to take them in a quiet room, alone, or with a teacher or aide present to provide structure and motivation, interpret questions, and manage time.

Alberto is an 11-year-old diagnosed with high-functioning autism. He is educated primarily in regular classrooms but receives some special tutoring in his school's resource room. In science class they were learning about species' classification, a topic that Alberto particularly enjoyed and was good at—his excellent memory helped him learn the Latin names and categories easily. His mother was therefore quite surprised when he brought home a test on animal classification with a large red F on the top. When she went in to talk to the science teacher, she found that the format of the test was very different from other tests, as well as from how Alberto and his classmates had learned and studied the material. Specifically, the teacher had given students a page of animal names that they were supposed to cut out and then arrange on a chart according to their species. While Alberto knew every name and classification by heart, he was not able to flexibly apply this knowledge to this new format. His mother demonstrated for the teacher how Alberto could fill in the blanks or answer short questions about every animal on the chart and how, in fact, he could even complete the chart once his mother explained the task to him and provided one example.

She then requested a new IEP meeting and had it written formally into Alberto's IEP that he be allowed to take tests for all his classes in the resource room, where the resource teacher could monitor his work and provide assistance and clarification when necessary. In addition, it was included in Alberto's IEP that his tests follow a standard format (specifically, fill-in-the-blank and short-answer questions). His mother and the resource teacher were also promised that they would be given advance notice of any test that would, of necessity, follow a different format so that they could teach Alberto how to respond in a different way and be sure he understood what was asked of him.

Comprehension and Abstraction Skills

Many children with Asperger syndrome or high-functioning autism will not exhibit any academic problems in their first few years of school. Parents may be told that the child is academically on a par with the other children or perhaps even more advanced than classmates in some areas. For some children, this advantage dwindles with time and they begin to fall behind classmates as the grades advance. This usually occurs because the concepts taught in school become progressively more abstract and require more interpretation, integration, and generalization than they did in lower grades. Thus, the strengths of most children with Asperger syndrome and high-functioning autism described in Chapter 5, such as memory and visualization, are highlighted in early grades, but progressively less required as the years go by. Conversely, the comprehension and abstraction skills that seem to be integral parts of the cognitive deficit profile of Asperger syndrome and high-functioning autism are increasingly required. What can be done to help your child with these kinds of skills?

Most of the answers to this question have already been provided somewhere in this chapter: make concepts as concrete and visual as possible, organize the work in advance, and use special interests or skills when you can. At the risk of some redundancy, we will provide some specific examples of how to use these principles to compensate for weaknesses in reading comprehension and math concepts.

Reading Comprehension. Capitalizing on the rule-following strength of AS-HFA, teachers and parents can teach rules for understanding stories. Especially in elementary grades, most stories have a common structure that includes four typical elements: (1) who, (2) did what, (3) and then, (4) the end. That is, someone (the "who" of the story) does or is involved in something (the "what"), which is followed by some resolution of the situation, and then an ending. Teachers can underline these elements in a story or highlight them in color-coded ink in advance. They can provide a list of questions in the same color ink, thus tapping into visual strengths to improve comprehension. Or they can ask students to generate alternate but plausible endings to the story or paraphrase the main points by retelling the story in their own words (pictures or a visual flowchart can be used to make this exercise as concrete as possible). Teachers need to be alert for rote or memorized responses that come straight from the story without true understanding (such as echoing sentences rather than restating ideas in the child's own words). Additional elements of story grammar, such as the location or setting ("where") and the reasons, intentions, or motives of characters ("why"), can be added as the child is able to handle them. But add the last item with care. It is so difficult for most AS-HFA children to judge the underlying human motives and interpersonal dynamics of a situation that they can get a reasonable handle on the rest of the story's structure only to be stymied by this one element.

Alex, a 16-year-old with Asperger syndrome, explained why he was failing 11th-grade English. "My teachers," he said, "are always asking me questions that they know the answers to, but I don't. Even when I try to figure out *why* someone did something in *The Scarlet Letter*, it's never the reason the teacher thinks they did it. I just have different ideas about things than they do. I especially hate to speculate why someone else did something. I can only say why I did something." Alex was fascinated with animals, especially endangered species, and was much better able to answer "why" questions about these topics than about Hester Prynne.

Math. As with reading (and much else in this chapter), improving comprehension of math concepts boils down to making the abstract concrete and visual. Whenever possible, students with AS-HFA should be allowed to use manipulative materials (rods, tokens, beans, and the like) to stand in for abstract concepts like addition, subtraction, multiplication, and division. They can be allowed to act out or draw pictures to represent the components in word problems. Critical aspects of word problems can be highlighted or color-coded in advance by teachers so that the student will recognize information pertaining to which mathematical operation should be performed or which variables should be attended to. To see how word problems correspond to mathematical calculations, students can make up their own word problems revolving around their special interests. For example, "7 – 5" becomes "If you had 7 Pokemon cards and lost 5 of them, how many would you have left?" There should be explicit practice generalizing math skills to real-life situations, as this often does not happen naturally. Toward that end, fractions can be practiced by learning to follow recipes, subtraction can be illustrated by calculating whether the appropriate amount of change has been received back from a fast-food purchase, and money concepts can be taught using catalogs of favorite items and menus from favorite restaurants.

Behavioral Issues

It may also be necessary for your school to set up a behavior plan or contract to deal with nonacademic challenging behaviors your child may demonstrate in school (such as interrupting, distracting others, constantly talking about topics of special interest, and aggression) that influence his or her education. Many of the behavioral interventions discussed in Chapters 4 and 6 can be helpful in the school setting, including frequently reinforcing desired behavior (perhaps using tokens or other systems), ignoring minor misbehavior, teaching the child self-management techniques, performing a thorough analysis of the function of the problem behavior, and supplying the child with alternative, more acceptable behaviors to achieve the same goals. Most special education teachers are trained in these techniques and use them with all their students, not just those with AS-HFA.

Transitions

Each new school year brings anxiety for both parent and child. The transition between elementary and junior high school is often a particularly scary time, because your child will now have to negotiate multiple teachers and classrooms. You may be able to alleviate some of this anxiety by planning a visit to the new school at the end of the summer to explore the building and begin to learn the locations of classrooms, locker, lunchroom, and bus stop. Your child may also need to practice his or her locker combination. You can ask the school to provide this in advance and then buy an inexpensive lock for home practice (it won't open, of course, to the same combination as the one at school, but your child can memorize the numbers and practice turning the dial in the appropriate directions). It may also be useful to ask school personnel to consider the physical layout of the building when scheduling your child's classes. They may be able to assign a locker that is relatively close to the different rooms or choose classes that happen to meet near each other, thus minimizing your child's travel time and the chance for confusion or tardiness. Provision of a school map with classrooms highlighted and numbered in the order in which the courses are scheduled can also be a useful visual tool.

Making transitions between teachers and negotiating their individual expectations and standards can also be difficult for the student with AS-HFA. One way to minimize this problem is to designate a supportive, central contact person such as a school counselor or resource teacher, who helps coordinate services, monitor progress, schedule meetings, and provide comfort and support to the child when needed. Ask to have such a coordinator designated as part of the IEP. If your school has an autism team, choose someone from this team. It is often best if this "go-to" person is someone other than a classroom teacher, because negotiating among the needs of the child, the desires of parents, the style of the teacher, and the constraints of the educational system can be very tricky.

Some Concluding Thoughts

Some of the problems described in this chapter could be eliminated if school personnel were educated regarding the learning style of students with AS-HFA. This education may start when you alert the school about your child's diagnosis. Some parents fear that sharing diagnostic information with educators will negatively "label" their son or daughter, resulting in substandard education or inappropriate reduction of academic and behavioral expectations. In our experience, this is rarely the case. In fact, as this chapter should make clear, a wide variety of special services, therapies, and accommodations can be provided in the school, at no cost to you or your family, that will help your child succeed in school. To access such services, however, you must make the specific nature of your child's academic needs known. This includes sharing diagnostic information and other test results that may be relevant. It may also mean steering interested educators and administrators to resources and information about Asperger syndrome and high-functioning autism. The Appendix at the end of this book includes some resources specific to the educational needs of students with AS-HFA that may be helpful to share with school personnel.

An important consideration is that your child's academic curriculum address functional and adaptive skills that he or she will need to be successful in later life. One of the most important outcomes of school for children and adolescents with mild AS-HFA is establishing good work habits, a positive self-concept, and independent living skills. This may mean that there will need to be considerable flexibility in designing your child's curriculum and an understanding that it may not follow the standard curriculum. Parents and teachers need to constantly ask, "Does this contribute to this child's long-term goals?" This is vastly more important than following a typical curriculum outline or worrying about the number of credits needed to graduate.

Finally, in keeping with a central theme of this book, it is always important to capitalize on your child's strengths to compensate for academic difficulties or areas of weakness in school. Many examples are already woven throughout this chapter. For example, supplementing oral directions with visual aids is a way to use your child's well-developed visualization skills to make up for one of his weaker skills. Similarly, giving your child written directions or written rules is a way to use his or her reading skills to maintain focus and teach more appropriate behavior. Your child's special interests can be used to motivate him or her in the classroom.

Joseph's teacher was considering using his interest in geography to counteract his growing boredom and disinterest in typical academic subjects. His parents proposed that subjects and skills taught to Joseph incorporate something related to geography whenever possible. For example, when the class was learning to make timelines in history, his parents asked the teacher to allow Joseph to make a timeline of explorers and their discoveries of different parts of the world. In science, when the rest of the class learned about the geology of Utah, Joseph was allowed to learn about the geology of his favorite country at the time, Brazil. In math, Joseph's teacher devised simple problems involving the mileage between different cities in Utah. And during reading, he let Joseph read any book he chose, rather than the one the class was reading together. In this way, his teachers and parents made positive use of his intense focus on geography, motivating him to work and rescuing his plummeting grades in all academic subjects. After seeing the success of this relatively simple intervention, Joseph's teacher added a geography unit for the whole class, even though it was not typically part of the third grade curriculum, and allowed Joseph to act as the "assistant teacher" during the module. He also asked Joseph to go to younger classrooms to read to children. This "special job" made Joseph feel important and good about some of his abilities, despite the teasing and other failures he was also experiencing at school. Helping others is often a very successful way to build self-esteem and self-efficacy.

Another way to use your child's talents to promote school success is to involve him or her in any school clubs or activities that use those talents or involve those special interests. Enroll your daughter in the computer club or the reading club. If your school doesn't have one already, volunteer to organize and run it. If your child has a natural talent for spelling, encourage him or her to participate in spelling bees. These activities will help integrate your child into the life of the school and help him or her feel like part of the school community rather than a peripheral member. Many other social issues raise their heads in the school setting as well—one of the most painful for parents is the teasing or bullying of their beloved son or daughter. It is to these tender issues that we turn our attention next, in Chapter 8.

CHAPTER 8

---

*The Social World of Children
and Adolescents with Asperger Syndrome
and High-Functioning Autism*

"Hello, Friend—Now Go Away"

Everyone diagnosed with an autism spectrum disorder has trouble with
social interchange, specifically with what we call *reciprocity*, the back-
and-forth interactions that make up all social encounters. In the very
remote, nonverbal children who have classic autism, reciprocity difficulties are obvious. In high-functioning children and adolescents with
AS-HFA, however, reciprocity problems may be more subtle. Parents
often describe a feeling of one-sidedness in interactions with their
child. Sometimes parents feel as if they must carry the whole relationship, supporting and scaffolding the interaction to establish some
meaningful connection. If they don't start the conversation or ask the
specific questions, the child may have very little to say or appear totally
content on his own. Other parents describe their child as having his or
her own agenda: the child either tells the parents what to do or talks on
and on without paying much attention to the parents or altering his or
her behavior in response to what the parents say or do.

When Seth starts talking about the stock market or the national
debt, there is no stopping him. During dinner, he likes to tell his parents about the NASDAQ's performance that day. After repeated at-

tempts to introduce other topics at the dinner table, his exasperated parents find themselves ignoring Seth when he talks about finances and carrying on their own conversation. They aren't sure whether to be worried or relieved that Seth barely seems to notice that they aren't paying attention and keeps talking. If they make a comment or try to add any relevant information, Seth pauses politely but then takes up where he left off, as if his parents hadn't said a word. His parents do consider this a small success, since just a year earlier Seth would become extremely upset whenever anyone made a comment and feel compelled to start anew, repeating every single thing he had said prior to the point of "interruption."

Social reciprocity problems may be even more evident with peers. Children and teens with AS-HFA are often described as "on the periphery." They often can be seen walking around the perimeter of the playground, uninvolved and seemingly uninterested in the boisterous play going on around them. They may demonstrate a strong need for control and insist that other kids follow their own rules. If peers balk at this, the child with AS-HFA may complain or express sadness because "other kids don't want to play what I want to play," but show little ability or motivation to negotiate or compromise.

Seth's parents often got reports from his teacher that Seth was "bossy" with other kids. They asked the school psychologist to observe Seth on the playground to collect some examples of this behavior, so that they would be able to work with him at home using specific situations and examples from the school day. The psychologist told them that Seth spent most of recess walking around the playground fence, talking to himself under his breath. When other children called out to him, Seth usually didn't seem to notice. Occasionally, he would reluctantly join games in progress. During the psychologist's observation, Seth accepted an invitation to play freeze-tag but then insisted that no one touch him and that he be allowed to be "it" immediately. He protested loudly and tried to hit the child who tagged him out. Seth eventually went back to the fence, where he began to drag a stick against it as he circled the playground's edge, far from the other children.

In structured settings, such as school or scout groups, some children or teens with AS-HFA may interact with other kids and even feel a bond with some of them, but few pursue these relationships outside these settings. For the few individuals with AS-HFA who do seek out other children outside prearranged situations, often there is still a relative lack of depth in the relationship. It may not be fully mutual, with one person being more committed to and interested in the relationship than the other. The relationship may be limited in focus, revolving primarily around a shared interest—for example, the kids may play video games side by side, but don't do anything else together. Or the friendship may not involve the same level of intimacy (for example, sharing secrets and feelings, relying on each other for support or help) as expected for a child of that age. Research studies show that many children with high-functioning autism and Asperger syndrome have a very limited concept of friendship. When asked what it means to be a friend, they give simple and concrete explanations ("someone who is nice to you" or "you play with them") and are much less likely than other children of the same age to mention qualities such as companionship, affection, selectivity, and trust.

Derrick, a young boy with Asperger syndrome, volunteered that he had many friends but then added poignantly, "Some of them are mean to me." Upon further questioning, it came out that Derrick considered anyone in his class whose name he knew to be his friend. Like many children with AS-HFA, Derrick was very vulnerable to teasing because of his social naivete and unusual style of relating to others. He recounted how earlier that day a classmate had given him a piece of candy; after he'd taken a taste, the child "informed" Derrick that the candy had "drugs" in it. Derrick spent the rest of the school day worried and crying.

How children and adolescents with AS-HFA react to their lack of friends and to peer rejection varies. Some desperately desire friends and feel left out and lonely. Others seem quite content; they either don't notice or don't care that they have no friends—they are truly "loners" at heart. Still others vary at different ages, in different settings, or from hour to hour, vacillating between feelings of loneliness and taking pleasure in solitude. Some adults in our social support group articulately describe a yearning for contact with others, but then only limited tolerance for brief interactions (summarized in one Internet chat room as "Hello, friend—now go away").

Social reciprocity problems are also evident in conversation. There may be very little back-and-forth, with domination by the person with

AS-HFA, who does not pick up on cues from the other person that he or she has something to say (as with Seth). The child with high-functioning autism or Asperger syndrome may not ask questions of others, particularly about their opinions, feelings, and experiences. The child may have difficulty keeping conversations going, particularly when direct questions are not posed.

Seth was playing on the sidewalk in front of his house with some action figures. A neighbor boy of approximately the same age came up and asked Seth where he had gotten the figures. Seth replied, "Disneyland," without looking up. The boy said excitedly, "Oh, I've been to Disneyland too!" Seth said nothing and the boy eventually walked away.

Many people with AS-HFA ask questions when they need to find out something but are much less comfortable making comments or "small talk." In fact they may have trouble with social chat and may rarely talk purely for social purposes.

Clint was in an elevator riding up to the fourth floor of the building in which his social support group took place. The group's therapist got in on level 2 and smiled at Clint. Last week's discussion in group had been about making small talk. One of the specific situations they had role-played was what to say during a brief interaction on an elevator. A few topics had been mentioned: perhaps the weather or the traffic. Clint decided to try something new. He said to the therapist, looking him directly in the eyes as he'd learned, "Gee, what's that terrible smell?" The therapist smiled politely, shrugged, and said, "I'm not sure. How was your drive down today?" Clint persisted, saying, "Boy, something really smells bad in here!"

John, another young man in the social support group, made this comment after a group discussion about conversation. "I know there is something called 'reciprocity.' I've heard of it. I know what the word means. I know it exists. I just don't understand it. I can't even identify it when it's happening. It's much like humans might feel about echolocation [of bats—this young man's interest]. We know echolocation exists. We just can't hear it, nor would we know how to understand it if it was within our auditory range. That's how reciprocity is for me."

Kids with AS-HFA tend not to use the same kind of social body language that others use. Their eye contact may be limited, they may not smile at the other person, their posture may not convey interest and attention, and they may not use socially encouraging gestures such as nodding. All of this can give the impression that the person with AS-HFA is not truly engaged in the conversation, is not listening, or is bored. Other problems sometimes seen in Asperger syndrome and high-functioning autism, such as aggression or an overly blunt communication style (sometimes interpreted as rude or offensive, although it is unintentional), can also pose a threat to social relationships. Even the special interests of individuals with AS-HFA contribute to poor reciprocity, because they are so focused and idiosyncratic that they are difficult for others to share (or the child doesn't actually *want* to share them, as with Seth). And there is very strong research documentation, in addition to many descriptions from parents, of lack of empathy and difficulty taking others' perspectives. All in all, kids with autism spectrum disorders often seem very self-centered. Although there is no intent to be selfish, and there is no malice behind their behavior, their social shortcomings can have a wide-ranging negative impact on their lives: in their relationships, on their academic and occupational success, and elsewhere.

Naturally, then, as parents you want to help your child or teenager learn to be a social creature in our social world. But how? If your son wants friends but can't make them, how can you help? What can his teachers do? What can you expect from a therapist? If your daughter seems to have little interest in friends, but needs to work on social behaviors so that she can someday live independently and keep a job, where can you turn for help? Strategies for improving social reciprocity in kids with AS-HFA follow.

Strategies for Improving Children's Social Behavior

Social skills can be taught in many different settings. The traditional arena is in a school or clinic, through an organized social skills group. However, as you shall see in this chapter, there are a variety of other places where and times when you can help your child acquire critical social skills: at home, around the neighborhood, and in nontherapeutic group settings (for example, scouts). Many of the principles and techniques used in typical therapeutic groups can be used by parents at home. In fact, social skills groups are much more beneficial if supplemented by follow-up at home. So whether your child attends such a group or not, it will be important for you to know what you can do outside the clinic to reinforce more appropriate social behavior too.

What Your Child's Therapist Can Offer

Group Social Skills Training

Your family may have adapted to your AS-HFA child's social deficits, and therefore you might not consider the problem an enormous one at home in your daily activities. But social difficulties tend to be more pronounced in groups and with peers. So social problems may in fact be fairly significant for your child at school, at the local playground, or in a scout troop. We know that people with AS-HFA have trouble generalizing from one situation to another, so it's important to teach social skills in settings that are similar to those in which the children experience difficulty. When teaching social behavior to a child with high-functioning autism or Asperger syndrome, the therapist or teacher may be impressed by how fast the child learns new skills, only to be surprised later at how poorly these skills are used with peers. Thus, teaching in a group context is essential.

Formal instruction, with specific skills taught sequentially, is also important. Most parents are not equipped to deliver this type of instruction, so you will probably have to look for a group at an outpatient clinic or school, where the therapy will be delivered by a therapist or teacher. This does not mean, however, that you're not part of the process. As managers of your child's care, you should think of yourselves as consumers of the social skills training that teachers and therapists can offer your child. If the group training offered to your child diverges substantially from what we describe here, in ways that seem unconstructive or counterproductive, you may want to look elsewhere for a different program or concentrate on other ways to teach social skills, outlined later in this chapter.

Unfortunately, there are currently very few published curricula to teach social skills to high-functioning children and adolescents with AS-HFA. Several social skills manuals for children with more general behavior or learning disorders do exist and can be helpful starting places for teachers or therapists wishing to design a curriculum for AS-HFA children (see the resource list in the Appendix), but often significant modifications are required to make the curriculum "autism-friendly."

As with interventions in the schools summarized in the last chapter, there are some basic principles for teaching social skills that capitalize on your child's strengths. We summarize these principles and give you examples of how they might be implemented in a therapy group in the box on page 192. Social skills training for children with AS-HFA should break down the complex social behaviors that most children learn automatically into concrete steps and rules that can be memorized and practiced in a variety of settings. Abstract concepts, like friendships, thoughts, and feelings, should be introduced through visual, tangible, "hands-on" activities as much as possible. For example, the therapist might hold a cardboard arrow at the side of your child's face, pointed at the person to whom he is speaking, to help him learn and practice eye contact. Written schedules use your child's natural reading abilities to help him or her transition from one task to another while minimizing anxiety. A predictable routine will capitalize on your child's memory and rule-following strengths to help him or her anticipate the different group activities. There should be a behavioral plan that specifies individual goals for group members and a specific system for delivering rewards. Social skills training will be difficult for your child and, as with all people, he or she may need to be enticed to participate in this less-than-favored and possibly very challenging activity.

A final important ingredient is collaboration with parents to promote generalization. Weekly therapy in a clinic will do little to change basic deficits of AS-HFA unless there is *daily* practice and reinforcement of the skills being learned in situations outside the therapy room. Thus, it is very important that you be aware of what your child is learning and that you be taught how to practice the skills or implement specific techniques at home, in the neighborhood, or at school. This may be accomplished partially through homework. It is also important that the therapists or teachers provide explicit opportunities to address the skills outside the group, in more natural settings for the child (for example, in the classroom, park, video arcade, bowling alley, or restaurant), perhaps through community outings. It is important that the teacher or therapist working with your child tell you how and where to

Basic Principles for Teaching Social Skills

Principle	*Examples*
Make the abstract concrete.	• Provide rules, such as "make eye contact for 5 seconds when you begin a conversation." • Break complex behaviors into steps, such as "a conversation consists of a beginning, a middle, and an end," and teach each step. • Use visual cues, such as a double-tipped arrow to depict the turn taking and back-and-forth of a conversation. • Use hands-on activities to practice, such as role-playing a conversation.
Help with transitions.	• Provide a written schedule that outlines the group activities in order. • Use a predictable routine every session, such as an opening discussion, a group activity, a role play, a snack, jokes, and good-bye.
Motivate.	• Set realistic goals for each child. • Provide rewards for attaining goals.
Generalize.	• Establish communication and collaboration between parents and therapists. • Give assignments to be completed outside the clinic, such as calling another group member and having a phone conversation. • Take outings into the community to practice skills, such as having conversations at a restaurant.

help your child practice away from the clinic or school. If this is not happening, request a private session with the therapist or group leader. Say that you want to be more involved in your child's therapy and request specific assignments or procedures for following up on skills at home.

A variety of topics should be covered in any social skills group for children and adolescents with Asperger syndrome and high-functioning autism. Perhaps most basic is teaching the nonverbal behaviors that are important to social interaction, such as appropriate eye contact, social distance, voice volume, and facial expression. We call this *social body language*. A typical program might also include the following topics:

- Friendship skills: greeting others, joining a group, taking turns, sharing, negotiating and compromising, following group rules, understanding the qualities of a good friend.
- Conversational skills: starting, maintaining, and ending a conversation; taking turns talking; commenting; asking others questions; expressing interest in others; choosing appropriate topics.
- Understanding thoughts and feelings: showing empathy, taking others' perspectives, handling difficult emotions.
- Social problem solving and conflict management: coping with being told "no," being teased, being left out.
- Self-awareness: learning about autism spectrum disorders, personal strengths, unique differences, and self-acceptance.

Cognitive-Behavioral Therapy

Another clinic-based therapeutic model that may be useful to teach social skills to adolescents and young adults with AS-HFA (those who are able to tolerate a bit more abstraction) is called *cognitive-behavioral therapy*. It was originally developed to help people with depression, who are often highly critical of themselves, pessimistic, and likely to interpret neutral events in a negative light (the "glass-is-half-empty" kind of person). At the crux of this therapy is showing people how their thoughts influence their feelings and how negative "self-talk" is related to (even causes) feelings of sadness and depression. The antidote, in a cognitive-behavioral therapy model, is to learn more positive self-talk, changing negative thoughts into positive ones and learning new ways of thinking about the self and the world. Cognitive-behavioral therapy turned out to be remarkably effective and is still a widely used treatment for depression and other psychological disorders.

Cognitive-behavioral therapy helps people focus on the causes and consequences of their behavior, as well as on the emotions and thoughts that accompany their behavior. Its relevance to people with AS-HFA should be readily apparent. Often, those with high-functioning autism or Asperger syndrome have trouble reading the social cues in the environment accurately, resulting in odd or unexpected behavior. They often report difficulty understanding their feelings and trouble differentiating among similar emotions. For example, some people with high-functioning autism or Asperger syndrome say that they can tell when they feel "bad" but are not sure if they are sad or angry and, most confusingly, aren't sure why. And they often have poor understanding of the consequences of their behavior. So cognitive-behavioral approaches may be of some use for the autism spectrum disorders.

Josh, a 15-year-old with Asperger syndrome, came to group one day and announced that he had had a bad week because he got expelled from school. When queried about the circumstances, he replied simply that he had pushed another boy's head into a water fountain. No other explanation was forthcoming, and Josh seemed almost puzzled by what had happened. The cognitive-behavioral model was used to help Josh and the other group members understand the links among situations, responses, and consequences. The group leader stressed the importance of four aspects of Josh's situation: *who*, did *what*, *when*, and *where*. Josh began with a simple description: "This kid made me mad at school." With the structural aid of a written list, he was eventually able to describe many specifics of the situation: details about the boy involved, what he had done (he called Josh "fatso"), time of day, and exactly where the incident had occurred. The group then explored three aspects of Josh's response: his emotions, his actions, and his thoughts (or self-talk). While he could readily identify his actions (shoving the boy's head into the water fountain), his emotions (shame, embarrassment, and anger) and especially his self-talk were murky to him. Finally, the group discussed both the short- and long-term consequences of Josh's response. Josh had a clear understanding of one consequence (his expulsion from school), but seemed to have very limited awareness of other outcomes of his actions (for example, that the other boy had been injured and that Josh might be more likely to be teased again in the future because of his extreme reaction). Using a cognitive-behavioral model significantly improved Josh's understanding of the situation and his ability to prevent a recurrence in the future. The group also addressed ways to change Josh's response, including substituting more positive self-talk, using relaxation techniques, and alerting a teacher when faced with teasing.

Cognitive-behavioral therapy, delivered in either a group or an individual format, may be helpful for teens and adults with AS-HFA, not only because of the mood problems that are so common in this group, but also because of the explicit links this therapy model makes among situations, responses, and consequences, concepts that are difficult for those with autism spectrum disorders. Cognitive-behavioral treatment is more structured and concrete than other forms of psychotherapy. Relying less on insight and judgment than other treatment models, it focuses instead on practical problem solving, making it an "autism-friendly" form of therapy. However, cognitive-behavioral approaches are probably too complex for most younger children with Asperger syndrome and high-functioning autism, so it is best to wait until adolescence and adulthood, when abstraction ability matures, to try this type of treatment.

Implicit Didacticism

At the University of Washington, some therapists are developing an approach called *implicit didacticism* that uses the therapeutic relationship as a forum for modeling and teaching social skills. This strategy aims to help people with AS-HFA learn appropriate social skills through the therapist's demonstration of appropriate social behaviors in realistic social settings, such as a cafeteria or a store. Through this combination of social modeling, personal accounts of social dilemmas and their resolution, and feedback about observed social behavior, the therapist teaches individuals with AS-HFA appropriate social behaviors and the art of picking up on social norms through observation.

Perry, an 18-year-old boy with Asperger syndrome, sees his therapist weekly for a traditional "talk therapy" session. Each week they review his highlights of the week, as well as any difficult experiences. His therapist reinforces the successful strategies he has used and suggests alternative strategies that may be helpful for similar scenarios in the future. The therapy also provides a context for the therapist to observe and provide input about his style of social interaction. When he is looking off into space or fiddling with a pencil, the therapist's comment "Gee, I must be boring, you're not even looking at me" can elicit more appropriate social behaviors that can be practiced and reinforced immediately. When Perry began college, his therapy sessions occasionally took place on campus, in social settings that he had to learn to navigate. For example, a therapy session took place in one of the university's cafeterias, where the therapist modeled for Perry how to order food, how to treat the cafeteria staff politely and congenially, how to pay, and how to bus his tray when he was done eating. Perry's family has noticed that the skills addressed in this psychotherapeutic format have carried over into both family interactions and Perry's dealings with peers.

Strategies for Teaching Social Skills Outside the Clinic

Earlier we stressed the importance of addressing social issues in a group setting, since this is where social problems usually arise, and thus this is where your child needs to practice social behavior. We also emphasized that you should practice and support your child's emerging social abilities at home whenever possible and that social skills training in a clinic alone would not do much good. In the following sections, we describe a variety of resources and techniques for working on social skills that can be used by anyone, across a variety of settings. These techniques will help your child improve his or her social behavior even when he or she is not within the four walls of the clinic or school, with a trained professional there to assist him. You are a key player in this endeavor. The following approaches do not require a professional degree to implement, just an interest in trying, a willingness to keep trying, flexibility, and a sense of humor. It is often helpful to initiate one intervention at a time so that you can monitor its success and get some sense of whether changes in the targeted behavior are occurring (and why). As always, it is useful to implement the intervention across settings whenever possible, to increase the rate of skill acquisition and improve the likelihood of generalization. And, should you run into any problems or need advice as you try any of these interventions at home, seek the help of an experienced autism spectrum disorders specialist.

Feedback and Modeling

Parents and siblings can be valuable role models for the child with AS-HFA. To be effective, however, you need to be very explicit and concrete about the skills you are modeling and about drawing your child's attention to them. You can do this in a variety of ways, but perhaps the most powerful is to videotape interactions for later review. This not only appeals to most children, all of whom like to "star" in their own movies, but also permits "real-time" provision of pointers. It is a more effective strategy to pause a video and highlight a problem or make a suggestion right at that moment than it is to try to reconstruct the situation later. Choose your battles—decide first what skill you want to highlight (for example, eye contact, turn taking, appropriate conversational topics, or sharing during play) and then focus your comments on that specific skill. Be sure to praise your child for things he or she is doing well (or even doing okay) and gently provide guidance in behaviors where he or she could improve. Try to phrase suggestions positively, giving examples of what your child can do to improve, rather than focusing on mistakes and using a lot of "don't" statements. It can sometimes be helpful to videotape siblings or peers engaged in similar interactions. Point out things those children did well ("See how Amanda is looking right in my eyes and nodding while I talk to her?") to explicitly draw your child's attention to the way the behavior is supposed to be performed. But also point out things that did not go smoothly in the interaction, so that your child with AS-HFA doesn't feel singled out or criticized unfairly.

Parents and siblings can provide a daily time to practice conversational skills at home, much as time is set aside for homework or piano practice. This might involve a 10-minute period each day in which you and your child talk in a structured manner. You may need to write down topics beforehand, to promote topic maintenance, avoid drifting to more preferred subjects, and help your child formulate some ideas in advance. You may want to use some visual aids, such as a cardboard arrow or spinner to indicate whose turn it is to talk or a script with suggested questions or comments. As just described, if you have a camcorder, you can videotape the conversations for later review and practice.

You may have been frustrated many times by the small amount of personal information that your child shares spontaneously with you. So it may seem ironic that you may also have to watch out for oversharing of personal information. When they decide to share, many children with AS-HFA don't know where to draw the line and end up creating an awkward situation for themselves and those around them. One young lady with high-functioning autism, who wondered about her sexual attraction to a classmate, suddenly began to explore this attraction aloud in the lunchroom. Many of her classmates felt "weirded out" by this sudden, excessive disclosure and started to avoid her. One way to prevent this situation is through the provision of very explicit feedback to your child. Most children and teens with AS-HFA do not catch on to subtle suggestions about behavior. Therefore, you need to be explicit in defining for your child which topics are appropriate and which are not, perhaps in the form of a list. Make sure your child learns to recognize some signs that the other person may be disinterested in or uncomfortable with what he or she is saying, such as looking surprised, trying to change the topic, or blushing, and then has a list of more appropriate conversational topics to revert to.

How to Get the Most Out of Clubs, Activities, and Play Dates

Just putting your child in situations with other children isn't enough to ensure that his or her social issues will be addressed. The suggestions in this section are a bit more focused than just enrolling your child in extracurricular activities that expose him or her to peers. Social groups, like scouts, can be helpful, but usually there must be some explicit structuring and specific interventions to make such situations beneficial. It may be more useful to choose some social group activity that revolves around your child's interests and talents, to make the experience palatable and to expose your child to others who are like-minded and therefore more inclined to accept and appreciate him. Many communities have computer, reading, or science clubs that may interest your child. If there is a university in your area, inquire about programs it may have for youth, which often revolve around similar themes.

Drama clubs can also be very helpful for children with AS-HFA. Your child may initially be self-conscious or otherwise reluctant to try such a group, but the benefits can be substantial. After all, what is acting other than being told what to say, how to behave, how to make your voice sound, and how to make your face look in certain social situations? We have seen several children with high-functioning autism and Asperger syndrome prosper in drama groups.

Although they may not be an adequate substitute for face-to-face social interaction, Internet chat rooms provide an excellent forum for mature older children, adolescents, and adults with AS-HFA to develop friendships and practice conversation. The anonymity associated with them and the absence of face-to-face contact can reduce anxiety in young people with AS-HFA, and the fact that many are organized around a common and explicit interest can be beneficial. In addition to enabling your child to practice conversation, chat rooms give him or her a chance to observe the conversations of others to provide models of social interchange. Internet chat rooms can also provide a sounding board for getting feedback on or normalizing "real world" social experiences and misadventures. There are also Internet chat rooms, such as #Autfriends (*autfriends.autistics.org*), specifically for people with autism spectrum disorders and those who care about them. Keep in mind that one downside of the anonymity of chat rooms is that little is known about the individuals with whom your child interacts. Therefore, you should be involved in friendships that develop in these forums and make the potential dangers of sharing personal information clear to your child.

If the situation is structured appropriately, parents can help guide younger children with AS-HFA through a "play date" and make it a successful learning experience. But don't stop with inviting another child over to play! It is important to choose an activity for your child and the friend to do together; don't rely on their ability to come up with something interactive. Many children would sit side by side and play video games the whole time. Choose an activity that requires some interaction, such as playing a board game, cooking a simple recipe, or working on an art project. Build in explicit social opportunities, such as giving one child the flour and the other child the measuring cups, or having each child decorate a cookie for the other person. This gives your child the chance to practice requesting, sharing, turn taking, and perspective taking. Be sure that the activity is appealing to both participants. *And* be sure that your child knows how to perform the requisite behaviors beforehand, perhaps by playing the game or making the recipe first with you or a sibling. Don't make learning the rules of the game part of the play date; have the goals of the play date be social, pure and simple. That is, have your child take existing skills and now use them with a peer. You may need to be present during most of the interaction, prompting and reminding both children about turn taking, sharing, negotiating, and the like. You may even find it helpful to use some visual aids to structure the interaction (such as a spinner to indicate whose turn it is, a recipe with pictures showing all the ingredients, or a written list of game rules). Your goal is to reduce your intervention and monitoring until the children can play together without adult assistance. This may take some time, but is more likely to happen eventually if you first provide structure than if you simply invite a peer to your home.

Keep in mind that most children—those with typical development included—need a lot of teaching and structure to have a successful playdate. Squabbles and difficulties sharing and accommodating to others are part and parcel of children's social development.

Social Scripts

Social scripts are nothing more than written prompts or guidelines for what to do and say in a common social situation. Although you may not be conscious of using them, most of us have a variety of social scripts in our repertoire that we use when faced with a specific social situation. For example, we all generally know what to do and say when we meet someone new: we might extend our hand, say hello, introduce ourselves, ask the other person's name, and so on. Most people also have a pretty consistent social script that they use when ordering food in a restaurant and when answering the telephone. People with AS-HFA, however, usually haven't constructed such social scripts or have them accessible. Thus, it can be very helpful to provide such a script, in a format conducive to how most people with high-functioning autism or Asperger syndrome learn (using written cues or other visual structure, for example). Given their typically good memory skills, children with AS-HFA may well be able to memorize components of the script so that the written instructions can eventually be dispensed with. Scripts are not difficult to write and require little more than putting yourself in your child's shoes and writing down the script you (or a child) would use in that situation.

Clint very much wanted to ask a woman he knew at work to a dance at his church, but he was very apprehensive about calling her on the telephone. His father reminisced about his own difficulty calling women for dates when he was a young man and suggested that Clint use a "phone script" that outlined the important things he needed to say. Clint warily agreed. His father wrote out the following script:

"Hello, is Cindy there please?"

"Hi, Cindy, this is Clint, from work." (*Pause until you make sure she knows who you are.*) "Am I catching you at a good time to talk for a moment?"

If no: "When could I give you a call back?" (*Pause for answer.*) "Okay, see you at work tomorrow. Bye."

If yes: "There's a dance at my church this Saturday evening. I was wondering if you are free and might like to go?"

If no: "Too bad. How about doing something else the weekend after? Maybe a movie?"

If yes: "Great. My dad will give us a ride. We'll pick you up at 7. What is your address?"

And so forth. Other examples of scripts you might provide to your child or teen include how to indicate uncertainty, ask for help, or buy something in a store. It is always best to practice the scripts several times with your child before expecting him to use them in public. Videotaping and reviewing the scripted interaction can again be extremely helpful.

The Social Skills Game

Stine Levy, a behavioral and educational consultant from Indiana, has developed a game to teach a variety of social skills to children with AS-HFA. This game is fairly easy for parents to adapt or construct at home. Using a game board similar to Candy Land or Monopoly, mark out spaces along a path and use color-coded cards to advance through the game. Different-colored cards require the players to do different things, including practice their social skills. For example, blue cards might indicate something fun to do ("Make a silly face," "Jump up and down twice," or "Pat your head while rubbing your stomach"). Yellow cards might be used for surprise twists in the game's rules ("Take another turn" or "Go back two spaces"). Green cards could be related to your child's special interest ("Name five planets" or "What is the capital of Kuwait?") or other fun topics ("What is your favorite TV show?" or

"Who do you know who has a pet dog?"). One color, perhaps red, is at the heart of the game and requires the child to perform some kind of social skill or make a social judgment (for example, "You want to watch a video, but your mom says no. What should you do?" or "You see a classmate at the grocery store who says hi. What could you say back?" or "Name two things you can do if someone teases you" or "Ask another player how his or her day was"). Red cards allow children to learn and practice social routines and scripts. The child's answers to the social questions on red cards can be written down in a notebook for later review. Prompting of more effective or acceptable strategies can be given when needed, thus providing another way to teach social skills that makes use of visual skills and structure, while also being fun.

Social Stories

Social Stories are written, sometimes illustrated, stories that present information about social situations. They were developed by Carol Gray, an educational consultant in the Michigan public school system (see the resources in the Appendix for more information). They are different from social scripts in being much less directive. Instead of just telling what to do and say, they supply critical information about the social situation, highlighting certain social cues and other people's motives or expectations. Most important, Social Stories provide a rationale for why the child should do or say what he or she is told to do or say. Carol Gray explains the need for such justification through the following example. If someone told us to go stand on our head in the corner, either we would refuse or we'd do it once (while the other person prompted and watched us) and then never again. Why? Because that behavior made no sense in that particular situation. It is much the same with our children with AS-HFA—we may tell them to do or say something that seems completely alien to them. So it is incumbent upon us to provide the *reason* behind certain social behaviors if we want our children to use them regularly. In fact, Ms. Gray suggests (and many researchers also believe) that this failure to understand the *"why"* of social behavior is at the crux of many of the difficulties associated with the autism spectrum disorders.

Ms. Gray outlines some very specific rules for writing an effective Social Story. For example, it should contain more informative statements (explaining social cues or providing reasons) than directive statements (telling the child what to do and say). Directives should be stated positively ("Do this" rather than "Don't do that"). It is outside the scope of this chapter to outline all the specific instructions for writing Social Stories; we refer you to the Appendix for additional resources if you are interested in these stories, which are widely used by parents in homes and are not difficult to design. Here is one example of a Social Story written to help a child learn appropriate behavior in the cafeteria at school.

Eating in the School Cafeteria

- When it's time for lunch, my teacher tells the class that it is time to go to the cafeteria.
- I walk to the cafeteria with all the other kids. I try to walk slowly.
- We have to wait in line for our food. I wait my turn to get my lunch. It is important to wait my turn. Other kids don't like me if I push ahead of them. I want other kids to like me.
- The lady behind the counter is very nice. She asks me what I want. I get to choose a main course, a vegetable, a dessert, and a drink. I point to each food, and she puts it on my tray.
- I can have only one dessert. If I have too much dessert, I might feel sick.
- I say "thank you" to the lunch lady.
- I push my tray to the end of the line and give my lunch card to the person at the cash register. She punches a hole in it. This hole tells them that I paid for my lunch.

Tracy, who has high-functioning autism and is 9 years old, had trouble with many aspects of the lunch situation. She didn't like to wait in line, she wanted to eat only desserts, and she cried and tantrummed when a hole was punched in her lunch card. The Social Story her parents wrote helped her understand *why* she needed to do these things. It also gave her some clear concrete rules she could follow. Her teachers put each bulleted item from the Social Story on a separate piece of paper, let Tracy draw a picture to illustrate each page, and allowed her to carry it on her tray at lunch. This intervention was very helpful in changing Tracy's cafeteria behavior, and her tantrums reduced dramatically almost immediately. Tracy's parents began making Social Stories to help her understand how to behave in many other difficult social situations, including being nice to her new baby brother, taking a shower, following mealtime routines, sitting still in synagogue, and riding an escalator at the mall.

Social Stories are thought to be helpful not only in providing justifications for social behavior, but also in being highly visually structured. They provide a written product that the child can refer back to at any time as a prompt or reminder. Social Stories can be written on index cards and taped to a child's desk to remind him or her of appropriate social behaviors in the classroom (raising hand, waiting in line, handling a change in class schedule, and so on). Many children keep their Social Stories organized in a notebook and enjoy rereading them with family or saving ones they no longer need as evidence of the progress they are making.

Narrating Life

The goal of Social Stories is to explain social cues and justify the importance of certain social behaviors to your child. There are other ways to accomplish this goal. One is a technique called "narrating life," developed by Linda Andron, a social worker at UCLA who specializes in helping individuals with AS-HFA. Dr. Brenda Smith Myles, a professor at the University of Kansas Medical Center, calls this approach "thinking out loud." As these names for the technique indicate, it involves providing a running commentary of your behavior and thought processes. For example, you can verbally describe what you are doing, why you are doing it, how you are making decisions, why you are selecting certain behaviors instead of others, and what cues you are noticing. This technique is quite a bit like a Social Story, but it is not visual, nor does it have a concrete product. This may mean that it will be less useful for some children, but its appeal is that it is incredibly simple to implement and can be used anywhere, at any time.

When Seth's mother went to the grocery store, she talked aloud to him as she performed every step of the process. As she chose a brand of soup, she said, "I think I'll buy this brand today. We've been having the other brand for so long that I think we're getting tired of it. Plus, this one is on sale." As she looked for a special item, she said aloud, "When I can't find something, I ask someone who works here. You can usually tell who is a store employee by their nametag." As Seth's mother chose which checkout line to stand in, she said, "This cashier looks fast and her line is pretty short. And she is smiling at everyone, so she looks friendly." As they waited in line, she said to Seth, "Sometimes it's hard to wait in such a long line. But it would be rude to push ahead, and others would get mad at me. And waiting gives me a chance to look at the magazines next to the checkout." As she opened her purse, she said, "Before we leave, I need to pay for all these things. If I don't have enough cash, I can use a check or a credit card." As they left the store together, his mother said to Seth, "That cashier sure was nice. I always like chatting with the cashier. If I can't think of anything to say, I mention the weather."

Friendship Files

Tony Attwood, author of *Asperger's Syndrome: A Guide for Parents and Professionals*, suggests that parents help their child create index cards that contain relevant information about peers. Keeping information about other kids' attributes, interests, and favorite activities in this format can make information easier to recall for your child and enable him or her to prepare in more concrete ways for interactions. Help your child use the cards to:

- Choose appropriate topics of conversation.
- Compliment others (through knowledge of their attributes).
- Choose activities that the peer might enjoy.

Friendship files thus not only promote friendship but, more broadly, teach your child important perspective-taking skills, such as being attuned to the interests of others and tailoring interactions around the partner.

Peer Coaching

A very different type of strategy that can be used to teach social skills is what we call *peer mediation*. What that means is that "typical" (non-AS-HFA) children of the same age interact in a more natural setting with children or teens who have AS-HFA . Just placing them in proximity to each other won't be enough (if your child is in any regular education classes, then this is already happening at school, and yet your child is still having social difficulties). Instead, the typical peers are explicitly taught how to initiate interactions, prompt social responses, give feedback, and reinforce children with AS-HFA. Often peer-mediated interventions are done in schools, but they can also be implemented in a clinic or community setting—they have even been adapted for use in the home (see below). Pioneers of this approach were researchers and special educators Drs. Strain, Odom, and Goldstein (see the Appendix for references).

In one peer-mediated approach, all children in an elementary school classroom (that happened to contain a child with AS-HFA) were taught "buddy skills," which included staying near the assigned partner, playing with him or her, and talking to the buddy. During "buddy time" (usually free play or recess) they were paired with another child in the class and taught to "stay, play, and talk" (for details of this and similar approaches and specific training regimens, see the Laushey and Heflin reference in the Appendix). Each day, the buddy pairs were rotated systematically, so that all children were paired with the child with Asperger syndrome or high-functioning autism, promoting generalization of the social skills across many individuals.

Dr. Catherine Lord, a researcher at the University of Michigan, has adapted some of these principles for use with older children and adolescents with AS-HFA (see the Appendix). She gives peers several simple guidelines for interacting with the person with high-functioning autism or Asperger syndrome, such as staying near them, joining their activity, making comments, praising them for even small interactive behaviors, and being persistent. General information about autism is shared with the typical peers. Possible situations (for example, the child with AS-HFA ignores the peer or talks on and on about reptiles) are role-played to give the typical peers some ideas about how to interact. After this, however, the adult does not serve as a therapist or interact directly with the children with AS-HFA, but instead lets the peers behave and interact with them. The therapists remain present to support, encourage, and protect the child with AS-HFA when necessary, but try to deliver the treatment through the typical peers, effectively eliminating themselves as the "middle man."

Research demonstrates that peer mediation approaches have clear benefits. One study showed that the rate of asking for things, getting another child's attention, waiting for a turn, and making eye contact increased two- to threefold after a peer intervention in a kindergarten classroom. It also appears that children with AS-HFA generalize new skills to other settings and maintain them well over time, probably because the need to transfer newly learned social skills from an adult therapist to same-age typical peers is eliminated.

You may want to approach your child's school to see if they would be willing to implement some type of peer-mediated intervention in the classroom. Or you may want to adapt this approach for use in your home, with siblings or neighborhood children serving in the role of the peer coach. If you do so, be sure to prepare and train the "peer" in advance. You know your child's particular quirks and social difficulties, so prepare the peer for problems that might arise and role-play how to deal with them. Give the peer a few rules to guide the interaction (for example, stay near John, keep trying to play with him, and ignore it when he talks to himself). Initially, monitor the interactions, much as described above in the section on structured play dates. Then step back and let the children interact.

Circle of Friends

This is an activity intended to help children who have few friends become part of a group and be included in social activities. It is best implemented in a classroom or other natural group setting (for example, scout camp or religious classes). A social "map" made of concentric circles is constructed, with the child at the center, the inner ring containing family, the next ring containing other supports (teachers, therapists, clergy), and the outer ring friends. In a classroom, a teacher might first construct a Circle of Friends for a few typical children. Then she constructs one for the child with AS-HFA. It becomes immediately apparent that the outer ring is visibly less dense relative to the typical peers, perhaps even empty. The teacher then asks for volunteers to be in the Circle of Friends of the child with AS-HFA. These volunteers are given a variety of assignments, from greeting the child when he enters the class, to engaging him in play or conversation on the playground, to sitting with him at lunch. The success of the Circle of Friends program appears to revolve around close monitoring of the "volunteer friends." Pretraining (much as is done with peer mediators in social skills groups, described above) is necessary. It should cover basics about autism, tips to engage the child, advice about what to do when unusual behaviors occur, and some role playing of potential situations. Once the intervention starts, short but regular (weekly) meetings are needed. The classroom or resource teacher or another school staff member should meet with the volunteers, listen to how they helped the child with AS-HFA that week, discuss problems that arose, and perhaps even role play or otherwise give suggestions for how to deal with the problems.

A similar intervention could be done at home, with neighborhood peers serving as volunteer friends. Working closely with the peers, giving them appropriate guidance and follow-up, is just as important if the Circle of Friends is constructed at home as it is at school. Be sure that the children you choose to become your child's friends are willing, eager, and well-armed with information about your child so that they can be successful.

Linda, Joseph's mother, decided to organize a Circle of Friends for him in their close-knit neighborhood. She contacted three of her neighbors who had children roughly the same age as Joseph, told them about the program, and asked them to ask their children if they would be willing to play. Two 8-year-old boys agreed to be in Joseph's Circle of Friends. They already knew Joseph around the neighborhood and therefore were aware of some of his quirks, but Linda decided to tell them more specifics about Asperger syndrome. She stressed that Joseph was very bright and told them of all his natural talents and special skills. She also told them that he sometimes had trouble knowing what to talk about and knowing when to stop talking. She role-played with the boys what to do when either of these situations arose. For example, when Joseph started talking about geography, she prompted the peers to say, "Oh, that's pretty interesting. Did you happen to see the Jazz game last night?" When Joseph started rambling, she taught the peers to hold up an index finger and say, "Whoa! Can I say something?," and then redirect the conversation in an appropriate way. She then gave each boy specific assignments, such as sitting with Joseph on the bus, riding bikes with him in the neighborhood cul-de-sac, and calling him on the phone. Linda checked in with the boys and their mothers by phone every week to see how things were going, if they had had any problems getting along, or had encountered situations that they didn't know how to handle. Linda hoped that the boys would genuinely grow to enjoy Joseph's company, but she decided that providing them with occasional treats, such as gift certificates to the video store and outings to the pizza parlor and video arcade would help them to remain committed to playing with Joseph. This was a lot of work for Linda, but the pleasure on Joseph's face when he got a phone call or was asked to come ride bikes was worth it.

Strategies to Improve
Your Child's Ability to Handle Emotion

One of the primary tasks of childhood is to learn to regulate emotional responses. For many children with AS-HFA, the process of emotional self-regulation is delayed and they are likely to need extra help learning to deal with strong emotions appropriately. For example, while most toddlers and many preschoolers regularly have tantrums when they are frustrated or don't get their way, by the time they enter elementary school most typically developing children have few or no tantrums. Older children and even adolescents with high-functioning autism or Asperger syndrome, on the other hand, may continue to have tantrums because they have not yet learned how to regulate their emotions. Obviously, this kind of behavior does not help them fit in socially and can be one of the causes of social rejection and isolation.

The most important aspect of emotion regulation is being aware of your body's internal states and the cues indicative of emotional arousal. For example, when a person becomes frustrated, his or her muscles may tense up. He or she may feel a hot rush of blood to his or her face and a sudden surge of energy. Being aware of and interpreting these physiological effects of emotional arousal is difficult for many children with autism spectrum disorders.

Andy's brothers loved going to the neighborhood arcade and often pestered their mother to take them there. She felt torn because Andy, a young boy with high-functioning autism, had such a hard time at the arcade. He enjoyed the experience at first, but he became so caught up in the flashing lights and sounds that he soon was out of control. He would giggle uncontrollably, run around wildly, and tackle other children. The outing inevitably ended in tears and felt like a disaster to all involved. Andy's brothers pleaded with their mother to leave Andy at home next time.

Tim, an adolescent with Asperger's syndrome, was a gifted student. Despite the fact that his arithmetic scores far surpassed his grade level, he had received several failing grades. His frustration threshold was so low that he frequently snapped in class when his pencil needed sharpening or he could not get the teacher's help quickly. He seemed unable to monitor the increasing tension in his body until it overtook him in a physical outburst, at which point he would throw his books and papers to the floor, scream "I've had it!," and march out of the classroom. The other students stared, whispered, and began to snicker.

In both of these examples, we see children who fail to monitor their level of arousal and encounter social difficulties as a result. There are a few strategies parents can use to help children learn to regulate their emotions better. First, you can encourage your child to use words to express his or her feelings. It is precisely when preschoolers learn to verbalize that their tantrums precipitously decrease. Begin by teaching your child to notice when he or she is experiencing an emotion, such as joy, anger, or sadness. Then verbally label these emotional states for your child and encourage your child to express these feelings in words (for example, "I am feeling angry!"). If your child needs it, you can also provide visual cues, such as a sheet of paper with several emotions depicted on it, to help your child figure out his or her emotional state (see the Appendix for resources).

After your child has expressed his or her feelings in words or by using pictures, provide some ways of coping with the emotionally arousing situations. At first you can make suggestions, even perhaps a list of coping strategies. For example, you can say, "If you are frustrated, you can ask for help or ask for a break or go on to a new problem." Eventually, however, you will want to ask your child to come up with solutions by him- or herself. Prompt your child to think of further alternatives to the strategies you have provided ("What *else* could you do if you get frustrated?").

Sometimes, however, your child's emotional state will be so strong that he'll need techniques to calm himself before he can discuss his feelings and ways to cope with them. One technique that is often helpful is called *progressive relaxation*. While your child lies prone and breathes deeply, verbally walk him through tensing (while breathing in) and relaxing (while exhaling) muscle groups from toe to head. As he becomes more comfortable with the process, you can teach your child to tense and relax the entire body quickly and subtly for use in stressful circumstances. An added benefit of this rapid relaxation technique is that the teaching process helps children better recognize the body states associated with tension and relaxation. A second calming strategy for your child is to engage in a relaxing activity, such as listening to music (a portable CD player can be helpful), chewing gum, drawing, having a back rub, or thinking of something comforting, such as a soft blanket or the fur of a favorite pet. A less direct strategy is to teach your child to ask for help or to remove herself from the situation when she becomes aware of potential overarousal. Tim, described above, might benefit from having a teacher's permission to leave the room for 2 minutes if he is experiencing frustration. Parents and teachers can facilitate this by providing clear places and plans for children to take a breather and specific signals or "break cards" to let others know they need time alone. Just knowing that this option is available may be helpful for your child with AS-HFA. Most children will benefit from using a combination of these strategies for learning and maintaining emotional control.

Dealing with Teasing and Bullying

Many children and teens with AS-HFA are teased, belittled, or bullied in school. The peer mediation approaches described above appear to foster greater peer acceptance, which may reduce the frequency of victimization by peers that can be a common part of the life of a child with AS-HFA. Peer buddies are especially useful to the child with high-functioning autism or Asperger syndrome during unstructured times of the school day, such as lunch or recess. It is well established that bullies rarely target a child who is part of a group (or even just in a pair); they tend to go after children who are alone and thus vulnerable.

There are several other techniques that have shown promise in reducing the likelihood that teasing or bullying will occur. Many approaches involve similar ingredients to those used in peer mediation programs, including providing information about autism to classmates and creating regular opportunities for interaction between children with AS-HFA and typical peers. Other programs involve assertiveness training and teaching the child specific techniques for standing up to bullies: asking for help, seeking out a safe teacher or place, walking away, using humor, and the like. If you have reason to suspect that your child is being bullied, contact your child's teacher and principal immediately. It is of the utmost importance that your child be protected, which means outlining specific plans to deal with different situations, establishing "safe" zones around the school, and better monitoring less-structured activities and situations where the harassment may take place. The resource list in the Appendix includes a variety of programs that schools and parents can use to stop bullying and create a safe environment for all children. Many schools are already implementing such programs due to the recent rash of school violence (none of which involved students with AS-HFA, but approximately two-thirds of which did involve children who were being bullied or teased).

The typical bullied child is insecure, anxious, and socially "adrift," with few friends or other supports. Children may also be teased because there is something different about them. This may well be the case with your child. In addition to the school-based solutions described above, you can help make your child more resistant to bullying by creating pride in the way he or she is different. A confident child is a difficult child to tease. Brent, a 10-year-old with high-functioning autism, was being taunted on the playground and called "virus boy" (due to his interest in viruses and bacteria). As his teacher later told it, Brent turned around and said, "Well, I like viruses because I have autism and because I have autism, I am much better at reading and video games than you." Brent, incidentally, had been enrolled in a social skills group that had emphasized these special strengths of autism. The bully was left speechless and walked away.

If unusual behaviors such as hand flapping, talking to him- or herself, or making noises appear to be the primary cause of your child's being teased, you might also try to help him or her become more aware of these behaviors and minimize their occurrence in public or when around peers. You might videotape your child and then point out instances of the behavior, teaching your child to identify the behavior reliably. As your child becomes aware of the behavior, you can institute a reward system (much like the self-management program described in Chapter 4) to decrease its occurrence. If the unusual behavior seems to serve a specific function, such as expressing excitement or alleviating boredom, more appropriate substitute behaviors can be taught—clapping instead of flapping or saying "Oh, yeah!" instead of making unusual noises—as discussed in Chapter 6.

Another way to help your child become aware of his or her differences, especially those that might lead to being teased, is through an explicit discussion about your child's diagnosis. As parents, you can talk with your child about the basic features of autism spectrum disorders, emphasizing whenever possible their special strengths and uniquely positive aspects. This can lead to a discussion of the unusual behaviors associated with the autism spectrum disorders and how they can put your child or teen at risk for teasing. A helpful metaphor in talking about ways people can stand out is that of gorillas and flamingos. "Gorillas" stand out because they display some highly noticeable negative behavior such as aggression and tantrums, while "flamingos" stand out because they are unique and interesting but very different from others. To the extent that your child does not want to stand out, you can help him identify and learn to monitor the behaviors that make him like a gorilla or (more often) a flamingo, using the techniques just described. You may also want to read personal accounts written by people with high-functioning autism or Asperger syndrome (such as Temple Grandin's *Thinking in Pictures*) or watch the movie *Rainman* together to make the characteristics of autism or Asperger syndrome more tangible and easier for your child to identify. There are also two books that may be helpful in introducing your child to his or her autism spectrum disorder: *I Am Special*, by Peter Vermeulen, and *What It Means to Me*, by Catherine Faherty (see the Appendix for more information). We discuss issues of self-esteem and self-identity further in the next chapter, which deals with issues specific to adolescents and adults.

CHAPTER 9

....

Looking Ahead
Asperger Syndrome and High-Functioning Autism in Late Adolescence and Adulthood

> I have braved raging winds.
> I have survived the strongest storms.
> I blew through the valley of paradise.
> I have been soaking wet.
> I have survived.
> I am who I am!
>
> *—An adolescent with*
> *Asperger syndrome*

Growing up presents a number of new challenges for children with AS-HFA and their parents. Junior high and high school bring a more complex and less structured educational environment, requiring the child with AS-HFA to make many more transitions, such as moving from class to class, and to develop greater independence and flexibility. The difficulties that children with AS-HFA have with organization and other executive function skills (discussed in Chapter 7) can make it especially challenging for them to achieve full independence. Social demands increase with age too. In early adolescence the desire to conform to social norms peaks, and this can be particularly hard for a child who is inherently a bit different from peers. This may be the first time, in fact, that many children with AS-HFA become aware of how different they are from other kids. On top of all these new demands, teenagers are expected to behave more maturely and to take on more complex social and emotional roles in relationships.

The Good News about Growing Older

Fortunately, adolescence and young adulthood have a plus side too. By this time, some people with AS-HFA, especially those who have received appropriate treatment for several years, have a solid set of tools for navigating social situations. Greater familiarity with the "rules" of social discourse can help them fit in and draw less negative attention from their peers than during childhood. At the same time, the typical adolescents and young adults around them are maturing too, which often means they are developing greater acceptance of differences in others. You can't count on tolerance, of course; cruelty among teenagers is widespread and well publicized, so you as a parent will want to continue to deal with any teasing and bullying of your child that does come up in the ways suggested in Chapter 8. But, in general, these sorts of problems do decrease in high school and drop to very low levels in adulthood.

There are no guarantees that this will work for your son or daughter, but eccentricities and idiosyncrasies can actually be a social asset in high school. Take Charles, for example. In grade school, his tendency to question authority and challenge the logic of rules frequently landed him in the principal's office. His constant disruptions of class to argue about a seemingly arbitrary rule or assignment annoyed his classmates and earned their scorn. But when Charles got to high school, he was suddenly surrounded by others who felt it was their duty to point out to authority figures the errors in their logic and the injustice in their expectations concerning students. Charles was still viewed as odd by his peers, but he was also a bit admired as the class maverick.

Another advantage of maturity is that in adulthood it becomes more acceptable to arrange one's social life around certain interests. Many typical adults socialize largely with coworkers, for example, and conversation often centers on office happenings or the subject of the work that they all have in common. For people with AS-HFA who have chosen occupations dealing with their particular interest, this means less talk about unfamiliar or uninteresting topics and therefore less social anxiety or discomfort. Because adults have limited leisure time, it's also very common for them to seek out people with similar interests, whether through clubs, over the Internet, or via other avenues. This, too, can help people with AS-HFA maintain a social life that is more rewarding than daunting.

Perhaps the most important advantage of maturity in adolescents with AS-HFA (as well as many typical teenagers) is that increased autonomy brings a greater opportunity to shape their own experience and seek a "niche" in the world that is more compatible with their own strengths and interests. Robin, a young woman with Asperger syndrome, was frustrated throughout childhood by others' lack of appreciation of her interest in photography. Her parents and teachers would continually try to get her to set aside this fascination to do schoolwork, and kids were always trying to escape her long speeches on photographic techniques. But in high school Robin gained both social stature and self-esteem when she joined the yearbook staff and found everyone hounding her for a chance to occupy some space in her viewfinder.

Because maturity brings the freedom to choose your own level and type of socialization, teens and adults with AS-HFA also have a wider range of social options than they did as children. Some—especially those who have had some social success and learned to find interpersonal interaction rewarding in itself—choose to socially "mainstream" themselves and stick with the path of "typical" socialization. For others, social activities still feel more uncomfortable than rewarding, and these young men and women may continue to favor solitary activities. If, after years of coaching in social skills, your child chooses a solitary path in adolescence, you may feel as if you've failed. Or you may worry that the happy adult life that was your ultimate goal for your child may never be reached. In that case, try to remember that whatever level of socialization your child is most comfortable with is the one most likely to make him or her happy. As a parent your job is to help provide your child with the skills to socialize, but ultimately it is his or her decision how to use these skills. All parents face the challenge of balancing what is best in their own eyes with the personal needs of their child. Most parents hope their child will lead a happy and productive life. It's important to remember that your definition of a happy and productive life may not agree with your child's, particularly in the area of amount and type of social contact.

Lauren, whom we first discussed in Chapter 1, had very little desire to socialize in high school. Her mother was terribly disappointed when she declined an invitation from a classmate to the prom. But when Lauren entered college, she met a "soulmate," another loner who was also majoring in physics and who shared her love of movies. She and this young man spent many weekend evenings together in the movie theater. When her mother asked what she and her friend talked about together, Lauren said, "Nothing." When her mother asked if they had ever gone out for dinner before the movie or if she had ever asked her friend in for a cup of coffee, she answered, "No." Lauren's mother tried to give her scripts and other support to take the relationship to another level. But over time it became clear that Lauren derived a great deal of satisfaction and pleasure from the relationship *as it was*. Her mother eventually could see, somewhat wistfully, that even though Lauren and her friend did not have a typical adult romantic relationship, she was content and far more social than she had ever been.

Another bit of good news about adolescence is that it may well be easier for your child with AS-HFA than you fear—and it may even be easier than it is for a typically developing child. Many individuals with AS-HFA are so comfortable with adults and so agreeable to rules that there is little of the rule breaking, limit testing, dangerous behavior, and questioning of authority that are so much a part of typical adolescence. We aren't saying that there won't be challenges, but it is fairly rare for the parents of teens with AS-HFA to have to face issues of green hair, body piercings, and drug use.

Critical Issues during Adolescence and Adulthood

Teenagers and adults with high-functioning autism and Asperger syndrome face many of the same challenges that they had to deal with in childhood. For parents, this means that the ideas you've been using to help your son or daughter will still help. Many, perhaps even most, people with AS-HFA continue to need support later in life, although the amount needed may well diminish over time. As you did when your child was younger, you should continue to play to his or her strengths whenever possible, capitalizing on excellent memory or visualization skills to make it easier for your maturing child to navigate higher education and the workplace. Most of the accommodations we recommended in Chapter 7 will continue to help in high school and college. Many of the tricks we offered in Chapter 6 to make home life easier will benefit your teen or adult child when he or she lives in a different residential setting. Most of the suggestions for easing social awkwardness and making friendships we discussed in Chapter 8 will still apply.

But, you may say, my child has just gone through a huge hormonal shift. She now has a job. The rest of the world's expectations are higher now that she is older. Can we really go on as if nothing has changed? In fact, some things do change for people with high-functioning autism and Asperger syndrome as they mature. You'll need to emphasize independence and functionality more than ever. You have to learn how to negotiate a new set of situations and settings so you can help your child do so. It becomes a bit harder to strike a balance between providing support and letting your teen or adult child struggle to figure things out for him- or herself. In this chapter, we'll help you understand when the changes you see in your child and the new struggles you encounter require a new approach.

As any parent of a teenager knows, adolescence is a challenging time. Naturally it is complicated by AS-HFA. In the following discussion we'll tell you how you can take your child's disorder into account in handling various adolescent social issues. Just as important, however, we'll try to help you see when it's AS-HFA that is causing your child to behave the way he or she is behaving and when it's adolescence itself.

You'll see in this chapter that we believe that your child will still need a good deal of support and structure. If this seems discouraging, please understand that much of what we know about adolescents and adults with high-functioning autism spectrum disorders comes from the study of individuals who were only recently diagnosed. These people have not had the benefit of the early and prolonged treatment that your child has probably had, and so naturally they require more structure and intervention than your child might, *if* he or she is quite high functioning and has had many years of intervention. As we continue to diagnose the mild autism spectrum disorders early, we will get an increasingly clear picture of what adults with AS-HFA who have had early intervention truly need. For now, however, you will need to sort through the following recommendations to figure out which are necessary for your teen or adult child. One way to do this is to see how far your child gets in education, career, and ability to live independently without the assistance of these recommendations. If your child seems unhappy or has failed to achieve at the level you believe he or she is capable of, some of the following supports probably will be needed. In our experience, continued intervention is necessary throughout the life of many people with high-functioning autism and Asperger syndrome.

Support People

As your child has grown, you (possibly with help from teachers and therapists) have served as facilitator, translator, and guide in a world that has often been difficult for him or her. You have been an advocate, doing whatever it takes to ensure that your child is provided with the services he or she needs. You've reinterpreted hundreds of mis-perceived social slights and smoothed over many inadvertent social faux pas. You have been a person to hug after a rough day at school and to extend a hand to high-five after a successful social event. Despite your incredible efforts and successes, with growing maturity your child needs to find support elsewhere. The more independent your son or daughter becomes, the less likely you will be there to assist.

Sometimes parents feel that they should take a less obtrusive role in the life of their child as he or she gets older. What seemed acceptable to help with at age 10 can seem infantile for a teenager. For example, perhaps you've walked your child to school every morning, but begin to wonder if that is still appropriate when he or she enters high school. Some adolescents with AS-HFA will continue to want this kind of support. Let your child's wishes dictate your behavior. Don't worry that your support and help will make your child look different or lead to ostracism by his or her peers. It is highly likely that all your child's classmates already know that he or she is different. Walking your child to school will not make that basic fact any worse and may make his or her life just a little bit easier and more comfortable.

But some teens with Asperger syndrome or high-functioning autism begin to demand independence from their parents and resent the support that they see as "interference." As we mentioned earlier in this chapter, this is usually a much less prominent problem than it may be for your typically developing teenagers. But if your teen with high-functioning autism or Asperger syndrome does begin to resent the support you are providing, you will have to figure out how to respond. Your teenager or young adult will likely still need advice, moral support, sympathy in times of difficulty, and shared joy after victories. How can you continue to provide the structure that you believe your adolescent needs, but in a way that will be accepted and that is constructive?

One way that you can back out of the support role as your child grows older is to recruit "helpers" in the community or the natural settings your child is encountering. Support may be provided by a friend, a case manager, a therapist, a coworker, or different people in different settings. Now, while your child is just entering adolescence, is the time to help your child understand the need to actively recruit people to turn to in times of trouble. Your child might end up needing continuing professional support, such as a job coach, but even if he or she does not, having support people in multiple environments will alleviate much of his or her anxiety.

John's mother was delighted that her son was joining the high school swim team. However, she also knew that locker rooms and team bus rides would present a host of confusing social situations for her son to decipher. She mentioned to John that she thought it would be a good idea for him to have a "go-to" person in case he became confused or uncertain in that setting. He liked the assistant coach and felt comfortable talking with him, so they agreed he was a viable mentor. Together they wrote a note describing how they would like him to be available for assistance. John showed it to him after practice the next week. The coach readily agreed. John found that over the course of the season his "mentor" was invaluable, helping him understand that hugging other teammates was appropriate only at certain times, that pointing out team fouls to the referee was unnecessary, and that several of the more colorful locker room quotes were better left unrepeated in the following day's recounting of the game.

John's mother's use of the term "go-to person" was quite intentional. When you discuss the need to identify support people ahead of time, it's important to respect your son or daughter's need for independence and self-reliance, as these are critical aspects of identity for any adolescent. Instead of using terms like "helper," employ "mentor" or "coach" to stress your child's expertise rather than to imply an absence of skill. Brainstorm with your child the many different situations where an "expert opinion" might be helpful, such as at school, in a job, or in an after-school club. Pick a person that your child would feel comfortable seeking advice from in each setting. To make things more official and to be certain that the support person is willing to accept this role, explain to the candidate that you would like him or her to be the person your child can approach with any questions or confusion in that setting, as John and his mother did. One young adult with autism worked out a similar arrangement with a supervisor at his place of employment. Whenever things got a little confusing and he wasn't quite sure how to handle them, he knew this person would be ready and willing to respond to his queries. In fact, this "go-to" person turned out to be so indispensable that a backup was selected in case the supervisor was unavailable.

Disclosure

If your child's symptoms lessen with age, as often happens, and if he or she branches out into new settings, the question of disclosure of your child's disorder will come up more and more often. At first you'll participate in the decision of whether or not to tell others that your child has AS-HFA. For example, it will be your call to determine whether or not to let the camp counselor, sports coach, or neighborhood parents know that your son or daughter has Asperger syndrome or high-functioning autism. Eventually, however, the decisions will be your child's to make, so introducing the issue and the decision-making process with him or her in early adolescence is good preparation. Your child will need to decide whether or not to disclose the diagnosis to employers and coworkers, friends and acquaintances, and perhaps even romantic interests in the future.

The pros and cons of disclosing will vary by context and circumstances, but you and your child should be aware that there are many benefits to sharing a diagnosis of AS-HFA and relevant information with people with whom your child will have contact. In many situations, like school, organized groups or sports teams, and work settings, disclosing the challenges of AS-HFA can help your child gain understanding from others or lead to special accommodations. It can head off misunderstandings about any unusual behaviors or perceived aloofness. It can even relieve the person of worry about having to conceal symptoms or about being on the fringes of the group.

Marcus paced across the foyer in his parents' home. Yesterday had been his first day at a new job at a computer company. For the first time, Marcus was working independently, without a job coach. Marcus is 22 years old and has high-functioning autism. He was worried that his behavior had come across as odd to some of his coworkers while he was being given a tour of the office. His mother noticed his anxious behavior and asked him what he was worrying about. When he explained the situation, his mother offered to hold a meeting in which she would explain his diagnosis to his coworkers. Marcus was initially resistant. He had worked so hard over so many years to overcome his diagnosis. His mother had an idea that was more acceptable to him. They worked out a short script that Marcus could use when he met a new coworker or was worried about an interaction. The script went like this: "I have a disorder called autism. Sometimes I'm not sure what to say or do in conversations and social interactions. I apologize if my behavior seemed rude. If you'd like to learn more about autism, I'd be glad to discuss it with you." Marcus had a great memory and had little difficulty memorizing the script. In the future, Marcus wound up using this approach to disclose his diagnosis to several of his coworkers. He was pleased to discover that they were open and accepting of this information and were eager to learn more and assist him in any way possible.

Despite Marcus's positive experience, there can be some risk inherent in disclosing as well. Disclosure may invite prejudice, especially since the image of classic, severe autism dominates much of society's understanding of autism spectrum disorders. There is even a chance, if your child's symptoms are subtle, that others may think he or she is making excuses for inappropriate behavior. But, in a broad sense, disclosing information about your child's diagnosis helps everyone with AS-HFA by normalizing the phenomenon and helping others appreciate how common the disorder is and how capable those with it can be. One rule of thumb we suggest is that if your child's differences would be obvious to others anyway, then providing an explanation for them by disclosing the diagnosis may well outweigh any perceived risks, such as stigma. On the other hand, if your child's symptoms have become so mild as to be mere "quirks" or personality traits that do not impair functioning, then disclosing the diagnosis may not be beneficial. Liane Willey, an adult with Asperger syndrome, has made the decision about disclosure many times and has included a number of important factors to consider in her book, *Pretending to Be Normal*, that you may also wish to access (see the Appendix for more information about this book). Also be aware that if there are substantial negative effects of disclosing the diagnosis in a work or educational setting, you may also wish to investigate your child's legal rights under antidiscrimination laws.

Once a decision has been made to share information about your teenage or adult child's diagnosis with others, together you must decide on an appropriate strategy to convey this information. This will no doubt vary according to who is being informed. For some individuals, like Marcus, a well-rehearsed speech is an appropriate first pass at disclosure. For others, it can be helpful to provide your child with cards, much like "business cards," that explain what AS-HFA is. These cards can be carried in a wallet, pocket, or purse and handed to another person in an awkward situation. For example the card might state, "I have Asperger syndrome. This is a disorder that affects my sense of social understanding, and sometimes I am uncertain how to behave or speak in social situations. Thank you for your understanding."

It is likely that many people, particularly those who will continue to have close contact with your child, will be interested in learning more about AS-HFA. You might provide these people with some literature about AS-HFA or some first-person published accounts, such as *Pretending to Be Normal* or *Thinking in Pictures* (see the Appendix). Another option, if the person is interested in devoting some time to gain a deeper understanding, would be to take the person to an AS-HFA meeting or conference. For individuals who wish to disclose openly and help others feel comfortable asking about AS-HFA, you might display relevant materials, such as books about AS-HFA, in a prominent place in your home. This opens the door for discussion but leaves whether to broach the subject to the visitor's discretion.

A more personal way to teach others about AS-HFA is to describe what it means in your own terms and share what the experience has been like in your family's particular case. This information can be conveyed via a medium comfortable for you or your child, such as a story, a poem, or a conversation. For most families with a child with AS-HFA, the decision to share additional information is a sensitive one. They would like to help others understand, but they are fearful of imposing or appearing pushy. We recommend making it clear to people that you

> *A disclosure card—or rehearsed script—can help your young adult with AS-HFA reveal the disorder:*
>
> "I have Asperger syndrome. This is a disorder that affects my sense of social understanding, and sometimes I am uncertain how to behave or speak in social situations. Thank you for your understanding."

have information and other opportunities for them to learn more about AS-HFA without making them feel obligated to learn about the diagnosis.

Sexual Development

Even parents with normal children often find sexuality a difficult subject to discuss, yet it's far too important a topic to avoid. Most adolescents between 13 and 18 report frequently thinking about sex, and 50% say they engaged in sexual intercourse before age 18. Adolescents with AS-HFA may lag in emotional or social development, but for many their biological drives develop on time. Given the reticence about personal matters so typical of those with AS-HFA, it is even more important for you than for a parent of a normal child to approach your child about this topic. Sometimes parents of children with AS-HFA wrongly assume that delays in social development and interests give them permission to delay conveying information about sexuality and puberty. We recommend, however, that you deliver this information on the same timetable, or even earlier, as you would for children without AS-HFA. In fact when it comes to discussing sexuality, it's not a question of *if* but of *when.* The answer, we firmly believe, is *early.* Don't put off this essential discussion until a crisis occurs. Important issues to address include sexual intercourse, birth control, nocturnal emissions, breast and testicular self-examination, masturbation, and menstruation.

Be specific and concrete in your discussions of sexuality with your child. Provide factually accurate information in a comprehensible and straightforward manner, perhaps referring to a book with illustrations. For example, set up a concrete system and schedule for hygiene related to menstruation. In addition to showing your daughter the materials she will need to use and how to use them, you might also want to furnish her with pictures or photographs showing the order in which each step is carried out. Be specific about how often she will need to change her pad or tampon. Allow her to use a watch with a timer, if necessary, or mark in her day planner when she needs to visit the bathroom. If your daughter's menstrual cycle is regular, mark the days on the calendar each month that she will need to carry supplies with her. Write out a script that she can use in class to ask to use the restroom.

Masturbation is another important topic to discuss with your adolescent. Masturbation is a natural means of exploring developing sexuality. Teach your child very specific rules in terms of when and where masturbation or the discussion of it is appropriate. One adolescent we know was so excited when he discovered masturbation that he began telling all of his friends about his wonderful discovery. His parents certainly wished they had thought to discuss the topic with him before he brought it up.

Since, particularly in adolescent boys, sexual arousal can be unpredictable but conspicuous, it is also helpful to work out a plan of action to help your child manage such circumstances. For example, you might tell your son that when he has an erection, he should remain seated or go to the restroom. One precaution to take when the teenage years of spontaneous erections approach is to make sure your child does not wear certain types of pants to school. Sweat pants, for example, can make sexual arousal extremely noticeable.

It's important not just to broach the subject of sexuality with your child but also to revisit it periodically to ensure that your child thoroughly comprehends the social rules surrounding sexuality. The best way to do so is to make sure that your child knows it is okay to talk with you about these matters. For a child who is not forthcoming, it may be necessary to approach him or her for an official update every few months. In a worst-case scenario, misunderstandings in this area could lead to individuals with AS-HFA becoming either unwitting sexual offenders or vulnerable to sexual victimization. If you find these topics too uncomfortable to broach, enlist the aid of a pediatrician, psychologist, or other health professional.

Romantic Relationships

Many parents have difficulty imagining a child with limited social interest eager to engage in intimate romantic relationships. People with AS-HFA vary greatly in their level of interest in romantic relationships. For some, interest in romance and sexual relationships develops along with physical sexual development, much as for their typical peers. For others, the complex emotional aspects of romance may delay interest in intimate relationships until late adolescence or adulthood. Some of our patients have developed romantic interests and later relationships or marriages. These relationships succeed when they are mutually beneficial—the partner with AS-HFA receives support and the typical partner gets a companion with remarkable honesty, faithfulness, and devotion. When they don't succeed, it is usually a consequence of the difficulties that people with AS-HFA have with emotional intimacy, intrusive interests and preoccupations, perspective taking, and compromise.

Other people with AS-HFA never develop an interest in romantic relationships. For many, such as Temple Grandin, the option of living a productive life without a partner is more appealing and less complicated. As a parent of a child with AS-HFA, your mentoring can help your child understand relevant issues and make informed choices in this area as an independent individual.

As your child develops sexual feelings, he or she will likely demonstrate sexual interest in others and develop a desire for intimate relationships. Recall your own experience of the anxiety that teenage romances provoked: the uncertainty, the confusion, and the bewilderment. For a child who has difficulty understanding more basic social interactions, these complexities of romance can be overwhelming. You can make this unfamiliar territory more comfortable for your child by providing concrete rules for dealing with people to whom he or she is attracted. Provide examples of appropriate and inappropriate behavior and how they might affect the person to whom they are directed. Your child may be highly motivated to do this exercise in perspective taking, because no one wants to make the wrong impression on the individual on whom he or she has a crush. Potential problem areas in which it is crucial to establish explicit guidelines include physical contact, staring, following, phone calls, visits, and types/topics of questions. Although few adolescents are adept at figuring out all the signals for returned interest or disinterest, this area may be particularly difficult for children with AS-HFA due to their difficulty in interpreting subtle social cues. Offer your child some basic guidelines for interpreting behaviors that may indicate mutual interest or a lack of interest. This will be important in ensuring that your child's romantic leanings do not cause others discomfort.

Angelo developed his first crush when he was 14. The object of his admiration was a sweet young woman named Ella. Although she understood that he had Asperger syndrome, and she liked him as a friend, she soon grew uncomfortable with his courtship. He would frequently interrupt her when she was in conversation with other people. She often felt uncomfortable because he gazed at her for long stretches of time. When she brought it to the attention of a school authority, Angelo was mortified and wanted to figure out what he was doing wrong. He and his parents drew up some guidelines to help him make sure his behavior was appropriate. They made clear that it was not appropriate to touch Ella, and they delineated situations in which it was not appropriate to approach her, such as when she was in midconversation or was reading in study hall. Looking toward the future, they made concrete rules (based on number of seconds elapsed) about what constituted staring versus casual eye contact. They also discussed some telltale signs that another person was or was not interested in one's advances. Angelo was disappointed that his relationship with Ella was not to be, but he looked forward to future romances.

Self-Awareness, Self-Esteem, and Identity Development

Adolescence may be the first time that children with AS-HFA begin to form an identity by pondering questions like "Who am I?" and "Where do I fit in?" and "What will I become?" These aspects of adolescent development pose a significant set of challenges for young people with AS-HFA.

One such area is definition of self-concept. Research suggests that boys and girls use different strategies to determine their own self-concept. For girls, self-concept often relates to perceptions of physical attractiveness. Young women with AS-HFA may find this problematic due to the close link between perceived attractiveness and social mastery and popularity. Among boys, physical prowess composes an important aspect of self-concept. Again, this presents a challenge for children with AS-HFA because of the common link between autism spectrum disorders and motor coordination problems (see Chapters 2 and 3).

Closely related to self-concept is self-esteem. Many adolescents experience periods of low self-esteem. Parents of children with AS-HFA can expect the same. Sources of low self-esteem among children with AS-HFA usually relate to wanting to be liked and to have friends but not knowing how to succeed.

Morality is another facet of adolescent identity development that is often problematic for children with AS-HFA. Although moral rigidity and righteousness can be a notable strength for children with AS-HFA, it can also cause some social difficulties. Superficially clear-cut moral guidelines can lead children to make poor judgments in adolescence, when interactions become more sophisticated and complex. Like many adolescents, children with AS-HFA may develop strong religious or political beliefs in response to these ambiguities. After reading a book on the meat-packing industry, one young woman with high-functioning autism decided that eating meat was unhealthy. In addition to simply changing her own diet, she attempted to influence others by pointing out to classmates and the school cafeteria staff all of the health dangers that the nonvegetarian menu items were likely to pose.

Problems with identity and self-esteem present a serious challenge to children with AS-HFA and their families, but there are several strategies you can use to deal with these issues. As we discussed in Chapter 5 and at the end of Chapter 8, emphasizing your child's strengths and special characteristics will help him or her develop positive self-esteem. For example, if your child has a great memory, you might jokingly refer to him or her as "Memory Master." Calling your child by this nickname when he demonstrates the skill makes clear that he has just done something special and gives him an easily referenced positive way of looking at himself.

Many teens and young adults with AS-HFA don't realize that their feelings of awkwardness and not fitting in are common and experienced at some point by almost everyone. Few people make it to adulthood without experiencing teasing and rejection. Help your child understand that this experience is par for the course. Sharing some of your own personal experiences during your teenage years can impress on your child that everyone experiences self-doubt as a teen and relieve some of the anxiety about herself that she may be experiencing.

There are also some published resources that were developed to assist in the exploration of self-identity: *I Am Special*, by Peter Vermeulen, and *What It Means to Me*, by Catherine Faherty (see the Appendix for more information).

Depression and Anxiety

During adolescence (and sometimes earlier), many children who were previously oblivious to or even content with their lack of social connections start to experience distress. In childhood, much of friendship consists solely of acting as "playmates" and engaging in activities, such as sports or video games, together. During adolescence, however, the very nature of friendship changes in several ways that can challenge young people with AS-HFA. Friendships become more sophisticated and complex, with an increasing emphasis on trust, mutual sharing of personal information, and common or admired personality characteristics. These changes in the nature of friendship often increase the social difficulties encountered by adolescents with AS-HFA. These problems are compounded by the burgeoning self-awareness and the ability to make comparisons between the self and others that develop during adolescence. Feeling excluded or irreparably different can and often does lead to depression among adolescents with AS-HFA. Real and perceived disparities with peers can lower an adolescent's sense of self-worth and promote a descent into depression. Anxiety disorders are also a common psychiatric disturbance experienced by teens and adults with AS-HFA.

Science has not yet clarified whether these mood problems result from the natural psychological consequences of managing AS-HFA or if they represent a biological disposition that is related to autism spectrum disorders. It may well be a combination of the stress of chronically trying to fit in, the pain of rejection, and a biological vulnerability to mood problems. Some research suggests that mood disorders run in the families of people with autism. Depression and anxiety disorders in family members usually appear well before the birth of the child with autism or Asperger syndrome, so they do not appear to be simply a reaction to the stress of raising a special needs child. Another piece of evidence is that the neurotransmitter serotonin (a brain chemical that helps brain cells communicate with each other) appears to be altered in individuals with autism spectrum disorders and individuals with depression. So AS-HFA and depression may co-occur so often for many reasons. Thus, you will need to be attentive to your child's mood and monitor whether the other interventions suggested in this book can remedy them. If not, you should consult a licensed clinical psychologist or an experienced child psychiatrist. Numerous forms of psychotherapy are appropriate for this variety of problem; there are also highly effective medications that can help your child through difficult periods.

Seizures

Another problem sometimes encountered during adolescence in individuals with autism spectrum disorders is the onset of seizure disorders. Approximately 25% of all individuals with autism spectrum disorders experience seizures, and adolescence is a time of particular vulnerability. In some cases, seizure activity is obvious, such as when your child loses consciousness and has violent convulsions of the entire body. In other kinds of seizures, however, the signs are less obvious. Your child may have short periods (maybe only a few seconds) in which he or she is unresponsive (doesn't respond to his or her name being called or to other things going on around him or her). Instead, he or she may stare off into space, blink his or her eyes repeatedly, or show some kind of unusual motor behavior (such as brushing the ground with the toe of the shoe repeatedly). If you suspect your child may be experiencing seizures, he or she should be screened by a neurologist using a clinical electroencephalogram. Most seizure disorders can be effectively treated with medication.

College

The benefits of high school, from approval for concentrating on a particular interest to tolerance for—even endorsement of—eccentricity, become even greater in college. There are also, of course, some significant difficulties. During college, many young people are on their own in ways they never have been before. Your less direct supervision over your child's academic performance may mean that his or her difficulties will be overlooked. The following are some compensatory strategies that we have found effective. Some of these tips are based on the account of Liane Willey, a college-educated adult with Asperger syndrome and author of the book *Pretending to Be Normal*. We suggest that you review the options for educational accommodations listed in Chapter 7 as well. Many techniques that helped your child in elementary and high school will continue to be beneficial at the college level.

Disclosing

You and your child will have to consider the pros and cons of disclosing we discussed earlier, but keep in mind that many potential sources of support in the college setting open up when students share their diagnosis with professors, advisers, and tutors. These professionals may have worked with other people with AS-HFA and can be an excellent source of guidance and support in this unfamiliar and often challenging setting. If your child feels uncomfortable disclosing, perhaps he or she could select one especially trustworthy person to disclose to, such as staff at the center that provides services for students with disabilities (available on all college campuses). This would ensure at least one support person on campus. Mental health professionals or others in the community might be viable alternatives if your child is hesitant to disclose to someone with direct academic connections. You can help decrease your adult child's discomfort with disclosure by normalizing the phenomenon. Let him or her know that there are hundreds, perhaps thousands, of other students on campus with disabilities, such as reading and attention problems. Most of these students do disclose their diagnosis to professors and make use of the services on campus for students with disabilities, which are legally mandated. For example, anyone with a recognized disability can usually take exams at the disability center, under quiet and less stressful conditions, and perhaps with extra time allowed.

Selecting Classes

Especially at first, when your adult child is acclimating to a new environment, advise and guide him or her to select classes that are well suited to his or her strengths and to bypass areas of difficulty. When

Ralph, a young man with autism, enrolled in college, one of the first classes he took was a philosophy class. He was a concrete thinker and had a difficult time with the subtle texts assigned. At times it was unclear to him why these questions were important to consider at all. He discussed his problem with his mother and decided to orient his schedule more toward classes that focused on concrete information and memorizing a lot of information. He sold his philosophy books and experienced academic success as a chemistry major.

You may even consider requesting that certain academic requirements that are especially difficult for many people with AS-HFA be waived. For example, foreign language study presents problems for many young adults with high-functioning autism and Asperger syndrome. Contacting the student disability center on campus is the best way to explore whether any of these requirements can be waived.

As we suggested in Chapter 7, your child may also want to enroll in small classes, where the amount of attention from the professor may be greater, or in less popular courses, where professors may be highly motivated to retain students.

Selecting Teachers

Review student evaluations and consult with other students to identify teachers who are well liked or known for their understanding and flexible personality. Empathic teachers may be more likely to help your child in times of difficulty. Many colleges publish course guides containing teacher ratings or make them available in the advising offices for each major to help make these decisions.

Requesting Accommodations

If there are specific ideas that could make the college experience more comfortable or less intimidating for your child, most colleges will gladly make accommodations to assist your child. Examples of accommodations that might be helpful for individuals with AS-HFA include being excused from group projects, receiving preferential seating to suit any auditory or visual sensitivity, and receiving advance notification for changes in schedule. Visual thinkers might ask professors to provide extra visual aids to help them process lectures and course materials.

Students with motor coordination difficulties might request extended time on written exams, oral exams, or the option of using a laptop or a tape recorder for note taking. Many colleges offer note-taking services to individuals with cognitive or physical characteristics that make note taking difficult.

Planning a Class Schedule

In planning a schedule, it's always better to start with too few classes than too many. For some students with AS-HFA, the transition to college is so challenging that a full course load would be overwhelming. Starting off slowly and building to a full schedule provides time to adjust to the many changes that college life entails. This will also provide your child with more time to complete work and to devote time to establishing social contacts and planning and engaging in social activities. As you help your child plan a schedule, keep in mind your child's sleeping habits. Try to avoid classes scheduled for an hour of the day when he or she is typically asleep or groggy. Keep a visual schedule posted in your child's room so he or she has a handy visual reminder of the times and locations of each class. Unlike high school, during college students are likely to have blocks of free time during the day. For individuals with AS-HFA who thrive on structure and routine, it is important to block these times out on the calendar and specify a designated purpose, such as study time, leisure time, or physical exercise. This added structure and predictability can make college life more comfortable for many people with AS-HFA and can reduce anxiety associated with transitions and changes in schedules.

Monitoring Deadlines

Keep a portable academic calendar with plenty of writing space to mark down homework due dates as well as dates related to registration and class drop deadlines. Encourage your child to check this calendar each morning to have a clear idea of the schedule for the day as well as any upcoming deadlines. Share important deadlines with your child's support people so that they can help him or her remember. Current technology, such as personal data assistants—especially those with automated reminders—can also help your child keep track of deadlines and schedules.

Promoting Study Skills

Consistency is crucial to good study habits. Again, planning specific blocks of study time and writing them into a schedule helps students remember to study and gives them a finite goal. These study sessions should be planned for a time of day when your child feels productive and alert. He or she should find a "study spot" in a library, student center, or computer lab that reliably offers peace and quiet. Students should experiment with different environments to find the type that best suits their own style. For example, some students might feel more comfortable in a dimly lit space with materials scattered around them, while others might prefer a bright, highly organized study spot. Within study sessions, your child might prefer to devote the entire time to one subject or to study several different subjects. If your child prefers the latter approach, it can be helpful to structure his or her time so that favorite subjects are studied last. This helps motivate your child to persevere through other topics and ensures that more challenging subjects will be addressed while energy is high and attention is most focused. Campus study centers or books on study skills can help out by providing study tips that are applicable to all students, including those with AS-HFA. Most colleges, in their center for students with disabilities, offer some sort of assistance to help students in the domain of organizational skills.

Promoting Social Opportunities

College will provide your adult child with numerous opportunities to further develop his or her social skills. There are many settings in college where social skills are taught at a more academic level. For example, classes in speech communication and drama emphasize how best to communicate, how to convey emotion, and how to read other people's response to you. Sociology and psychology classes can provide insight into the way others work and the "rules" underlying human behavior. An abundance of special interest groups, ranging from rock group fan clubs to star-gazing societies, provide opportunities for socialization within the comfort of an area of interest. Responding to the increasing presence of students with AS-HFA on college campuses, the administrative offices or student bodies of many colleges are developing autism spectrum disorder friendship or support groups.

Living Arrangements

Some families prefer to have their adult child with AS-HFA continue to live with them. Others, for various reasons, want their adult child to live in the community, in which case several different options are available. Some adults with high-functioning autism and Asperger syndrome are quite nervous about and uncomfortable with this idea, but many others want this opportunity. Many young adults see it as a way to "normalize" their experience by reaching the same milestone as their siblings and peers. A wealth of practical matters, such as housework, household maintenance, cooking, shopping, transportation, and bill paying, can make independent living difficult for individuals with AS-HFA, however. Your adult child's ability to accomplish these kinds of tasks *on his or her own, with minimal supervision,* needs to be considered when selecting the most appropriate living situation. If you're concerned about your child's ability to live independently, start at a more supported level; preparing your child for increased independence can make the transition less overwhelming. Remember, too, that none of these decisions are permanent.

Most outside-the-family-home living arrangements are accessed through state agencies (with the exception of the first one we discuss below, independent living). The first step in finding these living arrangements is determining your child's eligibility for these state services. The name of the agency that provides residential services differs from state to state, but it is usually the same agency that provides respite, vocational-rehabilitation, and other services to people with disabilities. Ask the doctor who diagnosed your child, your state autism society, or even your pediatrician for a referral. This agency should be listed in the "Government Pages" of your telephone book, under "State Government Offices." When you and your child begin the evaluation process that determines eligibility for services, be sure to emphasize the limitations your child has in accomplishing activities of daily life *independently*. Sometimes people with AS-HFA are denied state-funded disability services because their level of handicap is perceived as minimal compared to those with severe autism or mental retardation. But if you stress that your child cannot do necessary activities like feeding himself (since this requires shopping, money handling, and other skills he may not have) or engage in daily hygiene unless someone assists him, he will be more likely to be eligible for the residential assistance options we describe below.

Independent Living

Independent living refers to your adult child living on his or her own without professional or significant family support. Independent living might, however, include a roommate who could be a source of support. For adults with AS-HFA who are living independently, support people are especially crucial. Your child should have "go-to" people who live nearby and can be contacted for various kinds of support. People with AS-HFA who are able to live independently may still need professional help in areas that involve crucial decision making, such as selecting homeowner's or renter's insurance or life insurance, or in financial matters. Based on her firsthand experience living as an adult with Asperger syndrome, Liane Willey suggests some organizational strategies to help people with AS-HFA who are living independently. She also recommends that a support person help your adult child get these strategies up and running.

- Sort mail into color-coded bins according to type, such as magazines, bills, correspondence, and so on. Set a specific time on a certain day of the week to go through the bills bin and pay those that are due. This kind of structure and routine helps to ensure that bills will not be overlooked and deadlines will not be missed.
- Maintain color-coded files for documenting and storing information involving credit cards, automobile maintenance and insurance, checkbooks, family wills and related legal documents, financial records, home or life insurance, household appliance instructions and warranty information, and health records.
- Place a large dry-erase calendar in a prominent place in the house. Write in all household responsibilities or related appointments on a weekly or monthly schedule. It can be helpful to duplicate this information on a portable calendar or in an electronic organizer. In choosing these options, it is important to keep in mind the different strengths of these formats. Although a portable calendar is convenient because it can travel with your child,

it lacks the visual salience of a large calendar and is unlikely to be useful unless your child regularly pulls it out and examines it.

- For important one-time reminders, stick adhesive-backed notes on the bathroom mirror so they will be impossible to miss during the course of the day or when getting ready in the morning. Again, alarms on personal data assistants can be used as reminders.

For many people with AS-HFA, overwhelming sensory stimulation and crowds of people can make shopping extremely difficult. Thanks to catalogs and Internet shopping sites, however, your child may not have to leave home to obtain many items, including groceries. When your child does have to run errands or go shopping, ask a support person to go along. Or an adult child who finds certain errands less intimidating or enjoyable can offer to do those for a support person in exchange for the support person's taking over more challenging tasks for the person with AS-HFA.

Supervised Group Living

Another residential option that provides more support than independent living is supervised group living. One type of supervised group living is a group home, which is a residential facility for several individuals with disabilities. Group homes are usually houses in residential neighborhoods staffed by trained professionals who assist residents in areas like personal care, cooking, and housekeeping. Since group homes may serve individuals with various disabilities, it may be advantageous to seek one that specializes in autism spectrum disorders.

A second type of supervised group living is a supervised apartment. In a supervised apartment, an individual lives with fewer people, and professionals visit only a couple of times per week. This arrangement affords the residents more independence and greater responsibility and is therefore often an excellent means of preparation for independent living.

Skill Development Homes

In skill development homes residents live with a family in their dwelling and the family receives funding from the agency responsible for the

---

Tools for Growing Independence

- "Go-to" people in different settings: school, work, sports, clubs, social arenas.
- Disclosure cards or a rehearsed script.
- Explicit rules for romantic and sexual behavior.
- Visual calendars and personal data assistants with automated reminders.
- Exploration of autism, self-identity, and self-acceptance through books, support groups, and Internet chat rooms.
- Medication or other monitoring for mood problems.
- Educational accommodations in college.
- Mail-sorting systems and color-coded files for organizing paperwork.
- Internet shopping, such as grocery ordering and delivery services.
- Individualized Transition Plan to college or workplace.
- Internet business opportunities.
- Job coaches.
- Job procurement software and books.
- Residential living options through state agencies that determine eligibility.

---

individual's care. In this arrangement, the family members have been trained to work with people with autism spectrum disorders and can be expected to provide assistance and instruction in self-care skills and housekeeping.

Employment

Finding appropriate employment is crucial in many straightforward practical ways, but it is also an important means of boosting a person's self-esteem and providing social opportunities. You will want to begin planning for your child's eventual employment well before your child will actually approach the job market, probably as he or she enters adolescence. This provides time to prepare your child for the challenges of the workplace and to help him or her develop requisite marketable skills. Individuals with AS-HFA who have an IEP in school (see Chapter 7) are legally entitled to an Individualized Transition Plan beginning at age 14. This is mandated as part of the Individuals with Disabilities Education Act and the Americans with Disabilities Act, described in Chapter 7. The Transition Plan begins with an assessment, which can be formal, such as standardized testing to assess abilities and interests, or informal, such as input from family members or caregivers about the student's abilities. During this time, it is important to consider a variety of jobs in terms of desirability, appropriateness, availability, and accessibility. Skill development goals should be planned and should be matched to jobs that are likely to be available. Goals should include both teaching marketable skills and teaching workplace behavior. Job sampling is a means for students to gain work experience. It can help your child by allowing him or her to practice the new skills he or she is learning in school in an actual work environment. This will also assist your child by providing a clearer picture of his or her likes and dislikes and how they are related to particular aspects of the workplace or the job itself. Throughout the process of developing an Individualized Transition Plan it will be important to include a case manager or other support person who will be involved in assisting your child after age 21, when school systems will no longer be involved.

Employment Options

There are several different types of employment settings, discussed here in descending order of amount of independence and self-sufficiency required.

Competitive Employment

Competitive employment refers to the typical type of job that most people apply and compete for. Such jobs do not usually offer support for your adult child as part of the work environment, so they represent the most independent option of those we've listed. Some people with AS-HFA succeed in competitive employment, especially when they opt for jobs that play to their strengths (see below) or minimize the amount of interpersonal contact required. Also within the domain of competitive employment is self-employment, or running your own business. Although this can mean increased organizational demands, it also allows your adult child to make the rules and set things up to suit his or her own preferences or needs. It can also offer an opportunity to tailor employment to the person's own interests. People with AS-HFA may prefer the option of running a business over the Internet since it may reduce interpersonal contact and social demands. One young man we know ran a website that brokered the sale of used books.

Supported Employment

Supported employment refers to a system of supports that allow individuals with disabilities to obtain paid employment in the community. Supported employment includes individual placement, clustered or enclave models, mobile crews, and the entrepreneurial model. Individual placement refers to a model in which a specific job is developed for a specific person by a job coach. This professional also works with the individual on the job to help him or her develop the necessary skills to do the job well. The cluster or enclave placement model is similar, but the job coach works with a group of people at the employment site. Mobile crews also consist of a small group of individuals and one job coach, but they work at different job sites and for different employers (for example, cleaning homes or offices in the community). In the entrepreneurial model, a small business is developed to employ persons with disabilities. At Division TEACCH, the center for individuals with autism in North Carolina (described in Chapter 4), they have developed several businesses that are staffed by people with autism, including one that makes the materials needed for a test kit used by professionals to measure symptoms of autism.

Secure Employment

Secure employment refers to a facility-based employment placement in which an individual is guaranteed a job, usually doing basic tasks in a structured setting. In a secure employment setting, individuals also receive work skills and behavior training to prepare them for more independent and competitive work environments.

Sheltered Workshops

Like secure employment, sheltered workshops are employment services associated with training agencies that employ many individuals with disabilities. However, placement in a sheltered workshop setting may not provide sufficient training for individuals to progress toward more independent employment settings. For this reason, secure employment settings are generally preferable to sheltered workshops.

Choosing a Job

An appropriate job should play to the strengths of your son or daughter in terms of both preferences and natural abilities. We have discussed the passion and conviction with which many people with AS-HFA pursue their interests and the knowledge that they can accumulate about their preferred subject matter. Applying this enthusiasm and ability in the workplace is an ideal means of helping people with AS-HFA to succeed in employment. For example, a person who is fascinated by bus routes and schedules would be a natural candidate for a job with a transportation department. As we described in Chapter 5, a person interested in history might enjoy working in an archives department. Of course, there is more to successful employment than simply being interested in the job responsibilities. However, a passion for the subject matter addressed in the job can provide excellent motivation for confronting the challenges it presents.

Consider jobs that involve a high level of routine and order. "Rule-governed" people may be more likely to succeed in jobs that have clearly defined rules, procedures, or routines, such as in a payroll office, a library, or a business that performs data entry.

Rupert, an adult with high-functioning autism, worked in a small office building and delivered the mail to the individuals who worked there. He liked routine and was aware that he was able to perform better and more comfortably when things were as he expected them to be. With his supervisor, he set up a daily schedule and mail route. Sticking to this schedule and having an available "consultant" should things change helped Rupert to succeed in the workplace.

Look for job opportunities that capitalize on your child's strong visualization or memory skills. A great example of tailoring a job to a strength in visual thinking is Temple Grandin's remarkable ability to use her visual mind to construct and test cow-handling facilities. Employment opportunities that feature tangible tasks, such as cooking, organizing, or computer programming, seem naturally suited to people who tend to think in visual terms. Jobs that require knowledge of lots of specific details or facts, such as working with inventory or in a library, can be a good match for adults with AS-HFA who have a strong rote memory.

A useful place to begin is to compose a list of your child's likes and preferences. Think creatively. For example, an interest in crafts might be turned into a website where decorative items are sold. An interest in baseball could translate into trading and selling baseball memorabilia. It is important to consider such things as level of interpersonal contact, physical requirements, sensory stimulation and level of activity in the workplace, and the flexibility of the work schedule. Think about whether your child would enjoy or be able to tolerate these aspects of the work setting. Appropriate jobs might include engineer, computer programmer, florist, medical transcriber, artist/craftsman, musician, factory worker, architect, electronic repairperson, librarian, antiques/collectibles trader, and archivist. This is not by any means an exhaustive list. It is intended to provide a range of options, from those requiring advanced degrees to those that can be obtained fresh from high school, that all require good visual skills, involve high degrees of routine and order, and are more hands-on than abstract in nature.

There are also computerized resources to assist with job procurement. The Attainment Company (*www.attainmentcompany.com*) markets software for this purpose. At their website, you can peruse software that is designed to help you work through your child's characteristics and how they match up with job requirements and social skills associated with employment. The book *Asperger Syndrome Employment Workbook*, by Roger Meyer, an adult with Asperger syndrome, is also a helpful resource.

Especially for a first job, it is essential to pick one with a high probability of success. This will help your adult child adapt to the experience of working while reducing his or her worry about failure. It will also give your child a chance to experience at firsthand the reinforcing properties of succeeding in the workplace and earning a salary.

Interviewing

Interviewing is a crucial skill for all job applicants, so it's important to work specifically on this skill with your adult child. Make a specific and concrete list of inappropriate and appropriate behaviors. If you know of any inappropriate habits your child has, such as clearing her throat loudly or picking at scabs, include them on the list. Write out a script that includes likely questions that the interviewer will ask and appropriate responses. Practice this script with your child using role playing to help your child memorize answers and to increase his or her comfort in this type of situation. Be sure to pay attention to aspects of nonverbal communication in both the interviewer and your child. Important aspects of nonverbal behavior to include are greetings and good-byes, eye contact, voice volume and pace, display of emotion or anxiety, dressing appropriately, appearing well groomed, and proper posture. Emphasize to your child how important it will be to attend to everything the interviewer says during the interview. For more information about the types of behaviors that are helpful during interviews, consult a book addressing work application and interviewing particulars.

Once your child has practiced these skills and feels comfortable role-playing them with a support person, it can be helpful to do a "throw-away" interview. Apply for a job that will involve interviewing but is undesirable or in a less preferred field. Scheduling an interview with less riding on the line will give your child the opportunity to practice interviewing skills in a real setting. Doing so can reduce his or her anxiety and the feeling of total unfamiliarity when your child later interviews for a job he or she genuinely desires.

Workplace Accommodations

Before you can ask for accommodations in the workplace, your child must decide whether to disclose information about his or her diagnosis. Accommodations can be made in a number of areas. Adjustments in workspace may help with sensory or motor characteristics. Use visual approaches to teach job skills. Creating visual "supports" for the workplace, such as a written set of instructions or picture diagrams of the finished product, can be beneficial to visual thinkers. It may also be important to ask for special considerations if work requirements entail cooperating in groups. Scheduling accommodations could help increase routine or decrease unpredictability in work demands. Finally, it may be important to work out a plan with an employer for management and resolution of any crises that may develop on the job.

A Final Word

Our goal in this book has been to help you give your child the best chance possible for a full and happy life. As your understanding of the strengths associated with AS-HFA grows, so will your ability to conquer its challenges. And as you overcome the difficulties that your child's disorder presents, you will be more able to celebrate the gifts and joys that your unique son or daughter brings to your life. The challenges may never entirely go away, but with your understanding and proper treatment as early as possible, your child and family can expect lots of improvement over the years. The more we learn about Asperger syndrome and high-functioning autism, the more likely it is that your child will, in fact, lead a full and happy life.

APPENDIX

Resources

Books on Asperger Syndrome and High-Functioning Autism

General Information on Asperger Syndrome and High-Functioning Autism

Attwood, Tony. (1998). *Asperger's syndrome: A guide for parents and professionals*. London: Kingsley.

Baron-Cohen, Simon, & Bolton, Patrick. (1994). *Autism: The facts*. Oxford, UK: Oxford University Press.

Bashe, Patricia Romanowski, & Kirby, Barbara. (2001). *The OASIS guide to Asperger syndrome: Advice, support, insights, and inspiration*. New York: Crown.

Frith, Uta (Ed.). (1992). *Autism and Asperger syndrome*. Cambridge, UK: Cambridge University Press.

Gutstein, Steven. (2001). *Autism/Asperger's: Solving the relationship puzzle*. Arlington, TX: Future Horizons.

Howlin, Patricia. (1999). *Children with autism and Asperger syndrome: A guide for practitioners and carers*. New York: Wiley.

Klin, Ami, Volkmar, Fred, & Sparrow, Sara (Eds.). (2000). *Asperger syndrome*. New York: Guilford Press.

Mesibov, Gary B., Adams, Lynn W., & Klinger, Laura. (1998). *Autism: Understanding the disorder*. New York: Plenum Press.

Ratey, John, & Johnson, Catherine. (1998). *Shadow syndromes: The mild forms of major mental disorders that sabotage us*. New York: Bantam Doubleday Dell.

Schopler, Eric, Mesibov, Gary, & Kunce, Linda (Eds.). (1998). *Asperger syndrome or high-functioning autism?* New York: Plenum Press.

Siegel, Bryna. (1998). *The world of the autistic child: Understanding and treating autistic spectrum disorders.* Oxford, UK: Oxford University Press.

Waltz, Mitzi. (1999). *Pervasive developmental disorders: Finding a diagnosis and getting help for parents and patients with PDDNOS and atypical PDD.* Cambridge, UK: O'Reilly & Associates.

Wing, Lorna. (2001). *The autistic spectrum: A parents' guide to understanding and helping your child.* Berkeley, CA: Ulysses Press.

Parenting, Family Issues, and Parents' Perspectives

Andron, Linda. (2001). *Our journey through high-functioning autism and Asperger syndrome: A roadmap.* London: Kingsley

Brill, Marlene Targ. (2001). *Keys to parenting the child with autism* (2nd ed.). Hauppauge, NY: Barrons Educational Series.

Davies, Julie. (1994). *Able autistic children—children with Asperger syndrome: A booklet for brothers and sisters.* Nottingham, UK: University of Nottingham Press.

Fling, Echo. (2000). *Eating an artichoke: A mother's perspective on Asperger syndrome.* London: Kingsley.

Harris, Sandra. (1994). *Siblings of children with autism: A guide for families.* Bethesda, MD: Woodbine House.

Hart, Charles. (1993). *A parent's guide to autism: Answers to the most common questions.* Riverside, NJ: Pocket Books.

Hart, Charles. (1989). *Without reason: A family copes with two generations of autism.* Arlington, TX: Future Horizons.

Park, Clara. (2002). *Exiting nirvana: A daughter's life with autism.* Boston: Back Bay Books.

Powers, Michael. (2000). *Children with autism: A parent's guide* (2nd ed.). Bethesda, MD: Woodbine House.

Willey, Liane. (2001). *Asperger syndrome in the family: Redefining normal.* London: Kingsley.

Educational Issues

Blenk, Katie, & Fine, Doris. (1997). *Making school inclusion work: A guide to everyday practices.* Cambridge, MA: Brookline Books.

Cumine, Val, Leach, Julia, & Stevenson, Gill. (1998). *Asperger syndrome: A practical guide for teachers.* London: Fulton.

Fouse, Beth. (1999). *Creating a win–win IEP for students with autism: A how-to manual for parents and educators.* Arlington, TX: Future Horizons.

Fullerton, Ann. (1996). *Higher functioning adolescents and young adults with autism: A teacher's guide.* Austin, TX: Pro-Ed.

Gibb, Gordon, & Dyches, Tina Taylor. (1999). *Guide to writing quality individualized education programs (IEPs): What's best for students.* Boston: Allyn & Bacon.

Hodgdon, Linda A. (1995). *Visual strategies for improving communication: Practical supports for school and home.* Troy, MI: QuickRoberts.

Moyes, Rebecca, & Moreno, Susan. (2001). *Incorporating social goals in the classroom: A guide for teachers and parents of children with high-functioning autism and Asperger syndrome.* London: Kingsley.

Myles, Brenda Smith, & Adreon, Diane. (2001). *Asperger syndrome and adolescence: Practical solutions for school success.* Shawnee Mission, KS: Autism Asperger Publishing Co.

Myles, Brenda Smith, & Simpson, Richard. (1997). *Asperger syndrome: A guide for educators and parents.* Austin, TX: Pro-Ed.

Siegel, Lawrence. (2001). *The complete IEP guide: How to advocate for your special ed child* (2nd ed.). Berkeley, CA: Nolo Press.

Tanguay, Pamela, & Rourke, Byron. (2001). *Nonverbal learning disabilities at home: A parent's guide.* London: Kingsley.

Social Skills Training and Other Social Interventions

Antonello, Stephen. (1996). *Social skills development: Practical strategies for adolescents and adults with developmental disabilities.* Boston: Allyn & Bacon.

Duke, Marshall, Nowicki, Stephen, & Martin, Elisabeth. (1996). *Teaching your child the language of social success.* Atlanta: Peachtree.

Freeman, Sabrina, & Dake, Lorelei. (1997). *Teach me language: A social-language manual for children with autism, Asperger's syndrome and related disorders.* Langley, BC: SKF Books.

Garcia-Winner, Michelle. (2000). *Inside out: What makes a person with social cognitive deficits tick?* San Jose, CA: Winner Publications. (*www. socialthinking.com*)

Gray, Carol. (2000). *The new Social Story book, illustrated edition.* Arlington, TX: Future Horizons.

Gray, Carol. (1994). *Comic strip conversations.* Arlington, TX: Future Horizons.

Gray, Carol. (1993). *Taming the recess jungle.* Arlington, TX: Future Horizons.

Howlin, Patricia, Baron-Cohen, Simon, & Hadwin, Julie. (1998). *Teaching children with autism to mind-read: A practical guide for teachers and parents.* New York: Wiley.

Matthews, Andrew. (1991). *Making friends: A guide to getting along with people.* New York: Putnam.

Nowicki, Stephen, & Duke, Marshall. (1992). *Helping the child who doesn't fit in.* Atlanta: Peachtree.

Quill, Kathleen Ann. (1995). *Teaching children with autism: Strategies to enhance communication and socialization.* San Diego: Singular.

Quill, Kathleen Ann. (2000). *Do–watch–listen–say: Social and communication intervention for children with autism.* Baltimore, MD: Brookes.

Teasing and Bullying

Garrity, Carla, Baris, Mitchell, & Porter, William. (2000). *Bully-proofing your child: A parent's guide.* Longmont, CO: Sopris West.

Garrity, Carla, Jens, Kathryn, Porter, William, Sager, Nancy, & Short-Camilli, Cam. (2000). *Bully-proofing your school: A comprehensive approach for elementary schools.* Longmont, CO: Sopris West.

Garrity, Carla, Porter, William, & Baris, Mitchell. (2000). *Bully-proofing your child: First aid for hurt feelings.* Longmont, CO: Sopris West.

McCoy, Elin. (1997). *What to do when kids are mean to your child.* Pleasantville, NY: Reader's Digest Adult.

Romain, Trevor. (1997). *Bullies are a pain in the brain.* Minneapolis: Free Spirit. (This book is intended for children.)

Sheridan, Susan. (1998). *Why don't they like me?: Helping your child make and keep friends.* Longmont, CO: Sopris West.

Developing Self-Identity

Faherty, Catherine. (2000). *Asperger's ... What does it mean to me?: A workbook explaining self awareness and life lessons to the child or youth with high functioning autism or Asperger's.* Arlington, TX: Future Horizons.

Vermeulen, Peter. (2001). *I am special: Introducing children and young people to their autism spectrum disorder.* London: Kingsley.

Behavioral and Sensory Issues

Baker, Bruce, & Brightman, Alan. (1997). *Steps to independence: A skills training guide for parents and teachers of children with special needs.* Baltimore, MD: Brookes.

Durand, V. Mark. (1997). *Sleep better!: A guide to improving sleep for children with special needs.* Baltimore, MD: Brookes.

Kranowitz, Carol Stock. (1998). *The out of sync child: Recognizing and coping with sensory integration dysfunction.* Bellevue, WA: Perigee.

Myles, Brenda Smith, Cook, Katherine, & Miller, Louann. (2000). *Asperger syndrome and sensory issues: Practical solutions for making sense of the world.* Shawnee Mission, KS: Autism Asperger Publishing Co.

Myles, Brenda Smith, & Southwick, Jack. (1999). *Asperger syndrome and difficult moments: Practical solutions for tantrums, rage, and meltdowns.* Shawnee Mission, KS: Autism Asperger Publishing Co.

O'Neill, Robert, Horner, Robert, Albin, Richard, Storey, Keith, & Sprague, Jeffrey. (1996). *Functional assessment and program development for problem behavior: A practical handbook.* Pacific Grove, CA: Brookes/Cole.

Schopler, Eric. (1995). *Parent survival manual: A guide to crisis resolution in autism and related developmental disorders.* New York: Plenum Press.

Preschool Treatment Models

Greenspan, Stanley, & Wieder, Serena. (1998). *The child with special needs: Encouraging intellectual and emotional growth: The comprehensive approach to developmental challenges including autism, PDD, language and speech problems, and other related disorders.* Cambridge, MA: Perseus Press.

Harris, Sandra, & Handleman, Jan. (2000). *Preschool education programs for children with autism.* Austin, TX: Pro-Ed.

Maurice, Catherine, Green, Gina, & Luce, Stephen. (1996). *Behavioral intervention for young children with autism: A manual for parents and professionals.* Austin, TX: Pro Ed. (Describes the ABA model.)

Richman, Shira. (2001). *Raising a child with autism: A guide to applied behavior analysis for parents.* London: Kingsley.

Schopler, Eric, Lansing, Margaret, & Waters, Leslie. (1983). *Teaching activities for autistic children: Individualized assessment and treatment for autistic and developmentally disabled children.* Austin, TX: Pro-Ed. (Describes the TEACCH model.)

Adulthood and Employment

Howlin, Patricia. *Autism: Preparing for adulthood.* London: Routledge.

Meyer, Roger N. (2001). *Asperger syndrome employment workbook: An employment workbook for adults with Asperger syndrome* London: Kingsley.

Morgan, Hugh. (1996). *Adults with autism: A guide to theory and practice.* Cambridge, UK: Cambridge University Press.

Smith, Maria, Belcher, Ronald, & Johrs, Patricia. (1997). *A guide to successful employment for individuals with autism.* Baltimore, MD: Brookes.

Personal Accounts

Grandin, Temple. (1996). *Thinking in pictures and other reports from my life with autism.* New York: Vintage Books.

Grandin, Temple, & Scariano, Margaret. (1986). *Emergence: Labeled autistic.* New York: Warner Books.

Willey, Liane. (1999). *Pretending to be normal: Living with Asperger's syndrome.* London: Kingsley.

Newsletters

Advocate: Published by the Autism Society of America
http://www.autism-society.org

Autism Research Review International Newsletter
http://www.autism.com/ari/newslet.html

Connections Newsletter
http://www.connectionscenter.com/news.asp

Families for Early Autism Treatment Online Newsletter
http://www.feat.org/FEATNews/default.htm

The M.A.A.P.: A Quarterly Newsletter for Families of More Advanced Individuals with Autism, Asperger Syndrome, and PDD-NOS
http://www.maapservices.org

Videotapes

Ask me about Asperger's syndrome.
Michael Thompson Productions, P.O. Box 9334, Naperville, IL 60567

Asperger syndrome: Crossing the bridge.
with Liane Willey and Tony Attwood
Michael Thompson Productions, P.O. Box 9334, Naperville, IL 60567

Autism: Being friends.
Indiana Resource Center for Autism, 1991.
This videotape is an introduction to autism for elementary-aged children. It describes symptoms and gives tips for interacting with classmates with au-

tism. Helpful for classroom discussion or training peer buddies. To order: *www.isdd.indiana.edu/~cedir/pubcat.html*

Understanding Asperger syndrome.
Dr. Margot Prior, Department of Psychology, Royal Children's Hospital, Victoria, Australia; Phone: 03 9345 5881

Software

Attainment Company
http://*www.attainmentcompany.com*

Do2Learn
http://www.do2learn.com

LocuTour Multimedia
http://*www.learningfundamentals.com*

Mayer-Johnson
www.mayer-johnson.com

Scientific Learning
http://www.scilearn.com

Laureate Learning Systems
http://www.laureatelearning.com

Web Sites for Asperger Syndrome and Autism Resources

Asperger Syndrome Coalition of the United States
http://www.asperger.org

Asperger Syndrome Web Ring
http://aspie.freeservers.com/main.html

Asperger's Syndrome
www.human-nature.com/odmh/asperger.html

Autinet Forum
http://autinet.org

Autism Related Resources
http://quest.apana.org.au/~tlang/autism.htm

Autism Research Institute
http://www.autism.com/ari/

Autism Resource Network
http://www.autismbooks.com

Autism-Resources
http://www.autism-resources.com

Autism Resources
http://www.unc.edu/~cory/autism-info

Autism Society of America
http://www.autism-society.org

Autism Society of North Carolina Bookstore
http://www.autismsociety-nc.org

Autism Today
http://www.autismtoday.com

Bullying
www.nobully.org.nz

Center for the Study of Autism, Asperger Syndrome
http://www.autism.org

The Connections Center
http://www.connectionscenter.com

Do2Learn
http://www.do2learn.com

Families for Early Autism Treatment
http://www.feat.org

Future Horizons
http://www.futurehorizons-autism.com

MAAP Services, Inc.
http://www.maapservices.org/index.html

National Alliance for Autism Research
http://www.naar.org

National Autistic Society
http://www.nas.org.uk/

Online Asperger Syndrome Information and Support (O.A.S.I.S.)
http://www.udel.edu/bkirby/asperger/

Oops . . . Wrong Planet Syndrome
http://www.isn.net/~jypsy

Pervasive Developmental Disorders Web Site
http://info.med.Yale.edu/chldstdy/autism/

Special Needs Project: Good Books about Disabilities
www.SpecialNeeds.com

University of Washington Autism Homepage
http://depts.washington.edu/uwautism/index.html

Web Sites for Adults with Autism or Asperger Syndrome

The Asperger/HFA Association
http://home4.swipnet.se/~w-44675/english.html

Autism/Asperger's Syndrome Independent Living Association
http://www.amug.org/~a203/horse.html

Autism Network International
http://ani.autistics.org

Autistics.org
http://www.autistics.org

Cando
http://cando.lancs.ac.uk

University Students with Autism and Asperger's Syndrome
http://www.users.dircon.co.uk/~cns/

Web Sites for Families and Friends

Camphill Communities
www.camphill.org

Families of Adults Afflicted with Asperger's Syndrome (FAAAS)
http://www.faaas.org

Family Support
http:/www.patientcenters.com/autism/news/stress_family.html

Mothers United for Moral Support (MUMS)
www.netnet.net/mums

National Parent Network on Disabilities (NPND)
www.npnd.org

Planned Lifetime Advocacy Network
www.plan.ca

The Sibling Support Project
www.chmc.org/departmt/sibsupp

SibShops
http://www.seattlechildrens.org/sibsupp/

Support Groups

AAA: Autistic Adolescents and Adults
klbuckle@email.msn.com

#Asperger
http://www.inlv.demon.nl/irc.asperger/

Autinet Forum
http://www.autinet.org

The #Autism Channel
http://autfriends.autistics.org

Bay Area Asperger's Syndrome Information and Support
http://www.php.com/baasis.htm

Independent Living Forums (INLV)
http://www.inlv.demon.nl/

Mothers United for Moral Support (MUMS)
www.netnet.net/mums

National Parent Network on Disabilities (NPND)
www.npnd.org

The Sibling Support Project
www.chmc.org/departmt/sibsupp

The UK Autism Electronic mailing List
http://www.autism-uk.ed.ac.uk/welcome.html#began

Web Sites for Learning Disabilities and Other Disabilities

Association for Retarded Citizens (ARC)
http://www.thearc.org

Children and Adults with Attention-Deficit/Hyperactivity Disorder
http://www.chadd.org

LD in Depth: Learning Disabilities General Information
http://www.ldonline.org

Learning Disabilities Association of America
http://www.ldanatl.org

Nonverbal Learning Disability Line
http://www.nldline.com

Our-Kids: Devoted to Raising Special Kids with Special Needs
http://www.our-kids.org/

Medical Centers/Universities/Clinics

Autism Asperger Resource Center
4001 HC Miller Building
3901 Rainbow Boulevard
Kansas City, KS 66160
Phone: (913) 588-5988
Fax: (913) 588-5942

Bradley Hospital Developmental Disabilities Program
1011 Veterans Memorial Parkway
East Providence, RI 02915
Phone: (401) 434-3400

The Center for Asperger's Assessment and Intervention
The HELP Group
13130 Burbank Boulevard
Sherman Oaks, CA 91401
Phone: (818) 779-5262

The Center for Children with Special Needs
384-2 Merrow Road
Tolland, CT 06084
Phone: (860) 870-5313

Child Evaluation and Treatment Program
University of North Dakota
Altru Health System
P.O. Box 6002
Grand Forks, ND 58206
Phone: (701) 780-2477

The Connections Center
4120 Bellaire Boulevard
Houston, TX 77025
Phone: (713) 838-1362

Emory Autism Resource Center
Emory University
718 Gatewood Road
Atlanta, GA 30322
Phone: (404) 727-8350

Indiana Resource Center for Autism
Indiana Institute on Disability and Community
2853 East Tenth Street
Bloomington, IN 47408
Phone: (812) 855-6508
Fax: (812) 855-9630

Judevine Center for Autism
9455 Rott Road
St. Louis, MO 63127
Phone: (314) 849-4440
Fax: (314) 849-2721

Kennedy Krieger Institute
707 North Broadway
Baltimore, MD 21205
Phone: (888) 554-2080

Kentucky Autism Training Center
Weisskopf Center for the Evaluation of Children
911 South Brook Street
Louisville, KY 40203
Phone: (502) 852-4631 or (800) 334-8635 ext. 4631
Fax: (502) 852-7148

McLean Center for Neurointegrative Services
115 Mill Street
Belmont, MA 02478
Phone: (617) 855-2736

M.I.N.D. Institute
University of California–Davis
4860 Y Street, Suite 0101
Sacramento, CA 95817
Phone: (916) 734-6463

Schneider Children's Hospital
Developmental and Behavioral Pediatrics
Schneider Children's Hospital
269-01 76th Avenue
New Hyde Park, NY 11040
Phone: (718) 470-3540.

Speech/Language and Learning Services
626 120th Avenue, NE, Suite B201
Bellevue, WA 98005
Phone: (425) 556-6330
Fax: (425) 556-6325

Talk, Learn and Communicate
17535 15th Avenue, NE
Shoreline, WA 98155
Phone: (206) 440-9708
Fax: (206) 440-9774

Treatment and Education of Autistic and related Communication-handicapped
    CHildren (Division TEACCH)
University of North Carolina at Chapel Hill
CB #6305
Chapel Hill, NC 27599
Phone: (919) 966-5156
Fax: (919) 966-4003

UCLA Autism Clinic
300 Medical Plaza, Suite 1100
Los Angeles, CA 90024
Phone: (310) 825-0458

UCLA Neuropsychiatric Institute
760 Westwood Plaza
Los Angeles, CA 90024
Phone: (310) 825-0511

University of Miami Center for Autism and Related Disabilities
1500 Monza Avenue, 3rd Floor
Coral Gables, FL 33146-3004
Phone: (305) 284-6564; (800) 9-AUTISM ext. 2

University of Utah Autism Program
546 Chipeta Way, Suite 458 (Research Project)
Suite 441 (Clinic)
Salt Lake City, UT 84108
Phone: Clinic: (801) 585-1212; Research Project: (801) 585-9098

University of Washington Autism Center
Center on Human Development and Disability
Box 357920
University of Washington
Seattle, WA 98195
Phone: (206) 221-6806
Fax: (206) 543-5771

Yale Child Study Center Developmental Disabilities Clinic
P.O. Box 207900
New Haven, CT 06520-7900
Phone: (203) 737-4337

REFERENCES

American Psychiatric Association. (1994). *Diagnostic and statistical manual of mental disorders* (4th ed.). Washington, DC: Author.

Asperger, H. (1944/1991). "Autistic psychopathy" in childhood. In U. Frith (Ed.), *Autism and Asperger syndrome* (pp. 37–92). New York: Cambridge University Press.

Bachevalier, J. (1994). Medial temporal lobe structures and autism: A review of clinical and experimental findings. *Neuropsychologia, 32,* 627–648.

Bailey, A., Le Couteur, A., Gottesman, I., Bolton, P., Simonoff, E., Yuzda, E., & Rutter, M. (1995). Autism as a strongly genetic disorder: Evidence from a British twin study. *Psychological Medicine, 25,* 63–77.

Bailey, A., Luthert, P., Dean, A., Harding, B., Janota, I., Montgomery, M., Rutter, M., & Lantos, P. (1998). A clinicopathological study of autism. *Brain, 121,* 889–905.

Bailey, A., Palferman, S., Heavey, L., & LeCouteur, A. (1998). Autism: The phenotype in relatives. *Journal of Autism and Developmental Disorders, 28,* 369–392.

Baron-Cohen, S. (2000). Is Asperger syndrome/high-functioning autism necessarily a disability? *Development and Psychopathology, 12,* 489–500.

Baron-Cohen, S., Bolton, P., Wheelwright, S., Short, L., Mead, G., Smith, A., & Scahill, V. (1998). Autism occurs more often in families of physicists, engineers, and mathematicians. *Autism: The International Journal of Research and Practice, 2,* 296–301.

Baron-Cohen, S., Jolliffe, T., Mortimore, C. & Robertson, M. (1997). Another advanced test of theory of mind: Evidence from very high functioning adults with autism or Asperger syndrome. *Journal of Child Psychology and Psychiatry and Allied Disciplines, 38,* 813–822.

Baron-Cohen, S., Ring, H. A., Wheelwright, S., Bullmore, E., Brammer, M., Simmons, A., & Williams, S. (1999). Social intelligence in the normal and autistic brain: An fMRI study. *European Journal of Neuroscience, 11*, 1891–1898.

Baron-Cohen, S., Ring, H. A., Bullmore, E. T., Wheelwright, S., Ashwin, C., & Williams, S. C. (2000). The amygdala theory of autism. *Neuroscience and Biobehavioral Review, 24*, 355–364.

Bauminger, N., & Kasari, C. (2000). Loneliness and friendship in high-functioning children with autism. *Child Development, 71*, 447–456.

Bryan, L. C., & Gast, D. L. (2000). Teaching on-task and on-schedule behaviors to high-functioning children with autism via picture activity schedules. *Journal of Autism and Developmental Disorders, 30*, 553–567.

Bryson, S. E., Clark, B. S., & Smith, I. M. (1988). First report of a Canadian epidemiological study of autistic syndromes. *Journal of Child Psychology and Psychiatry and Allied Disciplines, 29*, 433–445.

Chakrabarti, S., & Fombonne, E. (2001). Pervasive developmental disorders in preschool children. *Journal of the American Medical Association, 285*, 3093–3099.

Cohen, D., & Volkmar, F. (1997). *Handbook of autism and pervasive developmental disorders* (2nd ed.). New York: Wiley.

Courchesne, E., Yeung Courchesne, R., Press, G. A., Hesselink, J. R., & Jernigan, T. L. (1988). Hypoplasia of cerebellar vermal lobules VI and VII in autism. *New England Journal of Medicine, 318*(21), 1349–1354.

Damasio, A. R., & Maurer, R. G. (1978). A neurological model for childhood autism. *Archives of Neurology, 35*, 777–786.

Dawson, G. (1996). Neuropsychology of autism: A report on the state of the science. *Journal of Autism and Developmental Disorders, 26*, 179–184.

Dawson, G. (1999). What are early indicators of risk for autism? *Journal of Autism and Developmental Disorders, 29*, 97.

Dawson, G., Carver, L., Meltzoff, A. N., Panagiotides, H., & McPartland, J. (in press). Neural correlates of face recognition in young children with autism spectrum disorder, developmental delay, and typical development. *Child Development*.

Dawson, G., Meltzoff, A. N., Osterling, J., & Rinaldi, J. (1998). Neuropsychological correlates of early symptoms in autism. *Child Development, 69*, 1276–1285.

Dawson, G., & Osterling, J. (1997). Early intervention in autism: Effectiveness and common elements of current approaches. In M. J. Guralnick (Ed.), *The effectiveness of early intervention: Second generation research* (pp. 307–326). Baltimore, MD: Brookes.

Eisenmajer, R., Prior, M., Leekam, S., Wing, L., Gould, J., & Ong, B. (1996). A comparison of clinical symptoms in individuals diagnosed with autism and

Asperger syndrome. *Journal of the American Academy of Child and Adolescent Psychiatry, 35,* 1523–1531.

Eisenmajer, R., Prior, M., Leekam, S., Wing, L., Ong, B., Gould, J., & Welham, M. (1998). Delayed language onset as a predictor of clinical symptoms in pervasive developmental disorders. *Journal of Autism and Developmental Disorders, 28,* 527–533.

Filipek, P. A., Accardo, P. J., Baranek, G. T., Cook, E. H., Dawson, G., Gordon, B., Gravel, J. S., Johnson, C. P., Kallan, R. J., Levy, S. E., Minshew, N. J., Ozonoff, S., Prizant, B. M., Rapin, I., Rogers, S. J., Stone, W., Teplin, S., Tuchman, R. F., & Volkmar, F. R. (2000). Practice parameters: The screening and diagnosis of autistic spectrum disorders. *Journal of Autism and Developmental Disorders, 29,* 439–484.

Fombonne, E. (1998). Epidemiological surveys of autism. In F. R. Volkmar (Ed.), *Autism and pervasive developmental disorders* (pp. 32–63). New York: Cambridge University Press.

Gerhardt, P. (2001). Employment: How to plan for your child's transition. *Advocate, 34,* 16–21.

Ghaziuddin, M., Tsai, L. Y., & Ghaziuddin, N. (1992a). A comparison of the diagnostic criteria for Asperger syndrome. *Journal of Autism and Developmental Disorders, 22,* 643–649.

Ghaziuddin, M., Tsai, L. Y., & Ghaziuddin, N. (1992b). A reappraisal of clumsiness as a diagnostic feature of Asperger syndrome. *Journal of Autism and Developmental Disorders, 22,* 651–656.

Gillberg, I. C., & Gillberg, C. (1989). Asperger syndrome—Some epidemiological considerations: A research note. *Journal of Child Psychology and Psychiatry, 30,* 631–638.

Gillberg, C., & Wing, L. (1999). Autism: Not an extremely rare disorder. *Acta Psychiatrica Scandinavica, 99,* 399–406.

Grandin, T. (1988). Teaching tips from a recovered autistic. *Focus on Autistic Behavior, 3,* 1–8.

Grandin, T. (1990). Needs of high functioning teenagers and adults with autism (tips from a recovered autistic). *Focus on Autistic Behavior, 5,* 1–15.

Gray, C. A. (1993). Social stories: Improving responses of students with autism with accurate social information. *Focus on Autistic Behavior, 8,* 1–10.

Gray, C. A. (1998). Social stories and comic strip conversations with students with Asperger syndrome and high-functioning autism. In E. Schopler, G. B. Mesibov, & L. Kunce (Eds.), *Asperger syndrome or high-functioning autism?* (pp. 167–198). New York: Plenum Press.

Happe, F. (1991). The autobiographical writings of three Asperger's syndrome adults: Problems of interpretations and implications for theory. In U. Frith (Ed.), *Autism and Asperger's syndrome* (pp. 207–242). Cambridge, UK: Cambridge University Press.

Happe, F., & Frith, U. (1991). Is autism a pervasive developmental disorder?: How useful is the "PDD" label? *Journal of Child Psychology and Psychiatry and Allied Disciplines, 32,* 1167–1168.

Herskowitz, V. (2001). Adult software offers life lessons. *Advocate, 34,* 28–31.

Howlin, P., & Goode, S. (1998). Outcome in adult life for people with autism and Asperger's syndrome. In F. R. Volkmar (Ed.), *Autism and pervasive developmental disorders* (pp. 209–241). New York: Cambridge University Press.

Hurlburt, R. T., Happe, F., & Frith, U. (1994). Sampling the form of inner experience in three adults with Asperger's syndrome. *Psychological Medicine, 24,* 385–395.

Kadesjo, B., Gillberg, C., & Hagberg, B. (1999). Autism and Asperger syndrome in seven-year-old children: A total population study. *Journal of Autism and Developmental Disorders, 29,* 327–331.

Kanner, L. (1943). Autistic disturbances of affective content. *Nervous Child, 2,* 217–250.

Klin, A., Volkmar, F. R., Sparrow, S. S., Cicchetti, D. V., & Rourke, B. P. (1995). Validity and neuropsychological characterization of Asperger syndrome: Convergence with nonverbal learning disabilities syndrome. *Journal of Child Psychology and Psychiatry, 36,* 1127–1140.

Kunce, L., & Mesibov, G. B. (1998). Educational approaches to high-functioning autism and Asperger syndrome. In E. Schopler, G. B. Mesibov & L. Kunce (Eds.), *Asperger syndrome or high-functioning autism?* (pp. 227–261). New York: Plenum Press.

Lainhart, J. E., Piven, J., Wzorek, M., Landa, R., Santangelo, S. L., Coon, H., & Folstein, S. E. (1997). Macrocephaly in children and adults with autism. *Journal of the American Academy of Child and Adolescent Psychiatry, 36,* 282–290.

Larsen, F. W. & Mouridsen, S. E. (1997). The outcome in children with childhood autism and Asperger syndrome originally diagnosed as psychotic: A 30–year follow-up study of subjects hospitalized as children. *European Child and Adolescent Psychiatry, 6,* 181–190.

Lord, C. (1995). Facilitating social inclusion: Examples from peer intervention programs. In E. Schopler & G. B. Mesibov (Eds.), *Learning and cognition in autism* (pp. 221–240). New York: Plenum Press.

Laushey, K. M., & Heflin, L. J. (2000). Enhancing social skills of kindergarten children with autism through the training of multiple peers as tutors. *Journal of Autism and Developmental Disorders, 30,* 183–193.

Lovaas, O. I. (1987). Behavioral treatment and normal educational and intellectual functioning in young autistic children. *Journal of Consulting and Clinical Psychology, 55,* 3–9.

Manjiviona, J., & Prior, M. (1995). Comparison of Asperger syndrome and high-functioning autistic children on a test of motor impairment. *Journal of Autism and Developmental Disorders, 25,* 23–39.

Marriage, K. J., Gordon, V., & Brand, L. (1995). A social skills group for boys with Asperger's syndrome. *Australian and New Zealand Journal of Psychiatry, 29,* 58–62.

Martin, A., Patzer, D. K., & Volkmar, F. R. (2000). Psychopharmacological treatment of higher-functioning pervasive developmental disorders. In A. Klin, F. R. Volkmar & S. S. Sparrow (Eds.), *Asperger syndrome* (pp. 210–228). New York: Guilford Press.

Mesibov, G. B. (1984). Social skills training with verbal autistic adolescents and adults: A program model. *Journal of Autism and Developmental Disorders, 14,* 395–404.

Miller, J. N., & Ozonoff, S. (1997). Did Asperger's cases have Asperger disorder? *Journal of Child Psychology and Psychiatry, 38,* 247–251.

Miller, J. N., & Ozonoff, S. (2000). The external validity of Asperger disorder: Lack of evidence from the domain of neuropsychology. *Journal of Abnormal Psychology, 109,* 227–238.

Mishna, F., & Muskat, B. (1998). Group therapy for boys with features of Asperger syndrome and concurrent learning disabilities: Finding a peer group. *Journal of Child and Adolescent Group Therapy, 8,* 97–114.

Nordin, V., & Gillberg, C. (1998). The long-term course of autistic disorders: Update on follow-up studies. *Acta Psychiatrica Scandinavica, 97,* 99–108.

Osterling, J., Dawson, G., & McPartland, J. (2001). Autism. In M. C. Roberts & H. Walker (Eds.), *Handbook of clinical child psychology* (3rd ed., pp. 432–452). New York: Wiley.

Ozonoff, S. (1998). Assessment and remediation of executive dysfunction in autism and Asperger syndrome. In E. Schopler, G. B. Mesibov, & L. Kunce (Eds.), *Asperger syndrome or high-functioning autism?* (pp. 263–289). New York: Plenum Press.

Ozonoff, S., & Miller, J. N. (1995). Teaching theory of mind: A new approach to social skills training for individuals with autism. *Journal of Autism and Developmental Disorders, 25,* 415–433.

Piven, J., Harper, J., Palmer, P., & Arndt, S. (1996). Course of behavioral change in autism: A retrospective study of high-IQ adolescents and adults. *Journal of the American Academy of Child and Adolescent Psychiatry, 35,* 523–529.

Rimland, E. R. (1964). *Infantile autism: The syndrome and its implications for a neural theory of behavior.* New York: Appleton-Century-Crofts.

Rogers, S. J. (1991). A psychotherapeutic approach for young children with pervasive developmental disorders. *Comprehensive Mental Health Care, 1,* 91–108.

Rogers, S. J. (1998). Empirically supported comprehensive treatments for young children with autism. *Journal of Clinical Child Psychology, 27*, 167–178.

Schopler, E. (1996). Are autism and Asperger syndrome different labels or different disabilities? *Journal of Autism and Developmental Disorders, 26*, 109–110.

Schopler, E., Mesibov, G. B., Shigley, R. H., & Bashford, A. (1984). Helping autistic children through their parents: The TEACCH model. In E. Schopler & G. B. Mesibov (Eds.), *The effects of autism on the family* (pp. 65–81). New York: Plenum Press.

Schultz, R. T., Gauthier, I., Klin, A., Fulbright, R. K., Anderson, A. W., Volkmar, F., Skudlarski, P., Lacadie, C., Cohen, D. J., & Gore, J. C. (2000). Abnormal ventral temporal cortical activity during face discrimination among individuals with autism and Asperger syndrome. *Archives of General Psychiatry, 57*, 331–340.

Schultz, R. T., & Klin, A. (in press). Social systems of the brain: Evidence from autism and related disorders. *Philosophical Transactions of the Royal Society,* Series B.

Siegel, D. J., Minshew, N. J., & Goldstein, G. (1996). Wechsler IQ profiles in diagnosis of high-functioning autism. *Journal of Autism and Developmental Disorders, 26*, 389–406.

Simpson, R. (1993). Tips for practitioners: Reinforcement of social story compliance. *Focus on Autistic Behavior, 8*, 15–16.

Sinclair, J. (1992). Personal essays. In E. Schopler & F. Mesibov (Eds.), *High functioning individual with autism* (pp. 289–306). New York: Plenum Press.

Sparks, B. F., Friedman, S. D., Shaw, D. W., Aylward, E. H., Echelard, D., Artru, A. A., Maravilla, K. R., Giedd, J. N., Munson, J., Dawson, G., & Dager, S. R. (in press). Brain structural abnormalities in young children with autism spectrum disorder. *Neurology*.

Swaggart, B., Gagnon, E., Bock, S., Earles, T., Quinn, C., Myles, B., & Simpson, R. (1995). Using social stories to teach social and behavioral skills to children with autism. *Focus on Autistic Behavior, 10*, 1–16.

Szatmari, P., Archer, L., Fisman, S., Streiner, D. L., & Wilson, F. (1995). Asperger's syndrome and autism: Differences in behavior, cognition, and adaptive functioning. *Journal of the American Academy of Child and Adolescent Psychiatry, 34*, 1662–1671.

Tantam, D. (1988). Asperger's syndrome. *Journal of Child Psychology and Psychiatry and Allied Disciplines, 29*, 245–255.

Tantam, D. (1988). Lifelong eccentricity and social isolation. *British Journal of Psychiatry, 153*, 783–791.

Tantam, D. (1991). Asperger's syndrome in adulthood. In U. Frith (Ed.),

Autism and Asperger syndrome. Cambridge, UK: Cambridge University Press.

Taylor, B., Miller, E., Farrington, C. P., Petropoulos, M., Favot-Mayaud, I., Li, J., & Waight, P. A. (1999). Autism and measles, mumps, and rubella vaccine: No epidemiological evidence for a causal association. *Lancet, 353,* 2026–2029.

Volkmar, F. R., Klin, A., Siegel, B., Szatmari, P., Lord, C., Campbell, M., Freeman, B. J., Cicchetti, D. V., Rutter, M., Kline, W., Buitelaar, J., Hattab, Y., Fombonne, E., Feuntes, J., Werry, J., Stone, W., Kerbeshian, J., Hoshino, Y., Bregman, J., Loveland, K., Szymanski, L., & Towbin, K. (1994). Field trial for autistic disorder in DSM-IV. *American Journal of Psychiatry, 151,* 1361–1367.

Wakefield, A. J., Murch, S. H., Anthony, A., Linnell, J., Casson, D. M., Malik, M., Berelowitz, M., Dhillon, A. P., Thomson, M. A., Harvey, P., Valentine, A., Davies, S. E., & Walker-Smith, J. A. (1998). Ileal–lymphoid–nodular hyperplasia, non-specific colitis, and pervasive developmental disorder in children. *Lancet, 351,* 637–641.

Warren, R. (1998). An immunologic theory for the development of some cases of autism. *CNS Spectrum, 3*(3), 71–79.

Wing, L. (1981). Asperger's syndrome: A clinical account. *Psychological Medicine, 11,* 115–129.

Wing, L. (1991). The relationship between Asperger's syndrome and Kanner's autism. In U. Frith (Ed.), *Autism and Asperger syndrome* (pp. 93–121). Cambridge, UK: Cambridge University Press.

INDEX

ABOUT THE AUTHORS

Sally Ozonoff, PhD, is an Associate Professor of Psychiatry on the faculty of the M.I.N.D. Institute, a national center for the study and treatment of autism spectrum disorders based at the University of California, Davis. Dr. Ozonoff has been working with and studying individuals with high-functioning autism spectrum disorders since 1985. She has published many papers on the diagnosis, causes, and treatment of Asperger syndrome and high-functioning autism, and has been funded by the National Institutes of Health to study these topics. Dr. Ozonoff serves on the editorial boards of three scientific journals devoted to autism and developmental psychopathology. Before moving to UC Davis in 2002, Dr. Ozonoff was on the faculty of the University of Utah for 11 years, where she directed the Autism Neuropsychology Laboratory and served on the boards of the Autism Society of Utah and the Carmen B. Pingree School for Autism in Salt Lake City. She was the codirector of the University of Utah Autism Specialty Clinic, where she enjoyed many hours working with wonderful and interesting people. She now lives in Davis, California, with her husband and two young daughters.

Geraldine Dawson, PhD, is Professor of Psychology and Director of the Autism Center at the University of Washington, which provides diagnostic and intervention services for children with autism spectrum disorders and their families. Dr. Dawson has had an active career as a scientist and clinician specializing in autism and the effects of experience on early brain development. She has written numerous scientific articles on these topics, and edited a number of books, including *Autism: Nature, Diagnosis and Treatment* and *Human Behavior and the Developing Brain*. Dr. Dawson has been the recipient of continuous research funding from the National Institutes of Health for her studies on autism and child psychopathology since 1983. She is well known for her pioneering research on early diagnosis and brain function in autism and early biological risk factors for psychopathology. Dr. Dawson has served on many national committees and task forces pertaining to child mental health, including scientific review and consensus panels of the National Institutes of Health. She has been associate editor for three scientific journals: the *Journal of Autism and Developmental Disorders*, *Psychophysiology*, and *Development and Psychopathology*. She is currently director of a multidisciplinary research program on autism spectrum disorders funded by the National Institutes of Health.

James McPartland received a bachelor's degree in psychology from Harvard University and is currently a doctoral candidate in the child clinical psychology program at the University of Washington. His clinical training has focused on diagnostic and treatment approaches with children with autism spectrum disorders. He is currently conducting studies on the nature of information-processing impairments experienced by individuals with Asperger syndrome and high-functioning autism.